LASIK

SECOND EDITION

A Guide to Laser Vision Correction

ERNEST W. KORNMEHL, M.D.

ROBERT K. MALONEY, M.D.

JONATHAN M. DAVIDORF, M.D.

ADDICUS BOOKS

OMAHA, NEBRASKA

An Addicus Nonfiction Book

ISBN 1-886039-79-8
ISBN 978-1886039-79-7
Second Edition

Cover design by Jack Kusler and Peri Poloni
Color illustrations by Mary Bryson
Black-and-white illustrations by Jack Kusler
Interior page design and composition by Stephen Tiano

This book is not intended to serve as a substitute for a physician, nor do the authors intend to give medical advice contrary to that of an attending physician.

Library of Congress Cataloging-in-Publication Data

Kornmehl, Ernest W., 1959-
    LASIK : a guide to laser vision correction / Ernest W. Kornmehl, Robert K. Maloney, Jonathan M. Davidorf.-- 2nd ed.
        p. cm.
Includes index.
    ISBN 1-886039-79-8 (alk. paper)
    1. LASIK (Eye surgery)--Popular works. I. Maloney, Robert K., 1958- II. Davidorf, Jonathan M.,1965- III. Title.
    RE336.K67 2006
    617.7'19059--dc22
                                                    2005035027

Addicus Books, Inc.
P.O. Box 45327
Omaha, Nebraska 68145
www.AddicusBooks.com
Printed in the United States of America
10 9 8 7 6 5 4 3 2 1

Contents

Acknowledgments

I would like to thank my wife, Ellen Kornmehl, MD, for her support of my efforts with this book; she is my role model for a caring, compassionate physician. I would also like to acknowledge my parents, Nathan and Frances Kornmehl, for teaching me that being a physician is a privilege and position of trust that can never be violated. I thank Melinda Jordan for her editorial help and for her assistance in developing a world-class laser center; I also wish to express my gratitude to the entire staff of the Kornmehl Laser Eye Associates for the extraordinary care they provide our patients. Finally, I am grateful to the thousands of patients, and the doctors who referred them, for entrusting me with their most precious sense—the gift of sight.

Ernest W. Kornmehl, MD

I wish to thank my father, who taught me to be uncompromising in the pursuit of excellence, and my mother, who taught me that great relationships require compromise. I particularly thank my fabulous wife, Nicole, for her patience with the demands of my chosen career. At times, she must wish that I had listened more to my mother's advice.

Robert K. Maloney, MD

I would like to thank my father, Dr. Bernard Davidorf, for introducing me to ophthalmology and my mother, Eleanor Davidorf, for teaching me the importance of listening to my patients. I also wish to thank my uncle, Dr. Frederick Davidorf, for encouraging me in my research endeavors and for teaching me the importance of communicating new ideas through scientific publication. I thank Dr. Roberto Zaldivar, my mentor in the field of refractive surgery. Most importantly, my deep appreciation goes to my wife, Jaime, and our three children, Carolena, Benjamin, and Oliver, for their energizing spirits, support, and understanding.

Jonathan Davidorf, MD

Introduction

Just about everyone knows someone who has had laser vision correction. That's not surprising when you consider that 9 million people have had LASIK in the United States. As the number of these procedures continues to grow, so, it seems, does the hype. Advertisements, articles, Web sites, and patient testimonials abound. Exciting as this technology is, there's a lot of misinformation that can be confusing to those considering laser vision correction.

Why, for example, does one center offer laser vision correction for half the price of another center? And what is the consumer to make of ads claiming you can "throw your eyeglasses away for good!" and "get 20/20 vision—guaranteed"? A smart consumer considering laser vision correction needs to become well-informed. It is essential that you arm yourself with unbiased, complete information before undergoing such a procedure.

That's why we embarked on writing this book: to provide you with an easy to understand, thorough, and accurate educational tool that will answer your questions about one of the most popular surgical procedures—LASIK vision correction. We are committed to helping people understand the real—not the hyped—benefits of LASIK, as well as its disadvantages and potential risks.

If you are contemplating laser vision correction, you will want to know whether you are a good candidate for LASIK. You will need to find out exactly what is involved, how the procedure works, and how much it costs. You will also want to know what kind of eyesight you can reasonably expect after the surgery, as well as all the possible risks and complications. And you may need guidance on choosing a qualified laser surgeon—someone you can really trust. It is our intent to provide this kind of information in our book.

In our medical practices, we collectively have performed more than 65,000 LASIK procedures, and we talk to thousands of patients each year. When it comes to LASIK, similar questions come up again and again. We kept these questions in mind as we worked on this book. We also understand the kinds of anxieties and misconceptions most patients have when they enter our offices for the first time. We wrote this book to give you the benefit of our experience of having taken care of tens of thousands of patients. It is our hope that we can relieve your fears by thoroughly educating you about LASIK.

1

The Human Eye and How Vision Works

S ight is our most precious sense. Our eyes enable us to take in the surrounding world. Without sight, the way we perceive the world would be forever changed. No wonder the eyes are often elevated in literature, art, religion, and philosophy to symbolize everything from the windows of the soul to supreme wisdom. Indeed, the eyes are a marvel of mechanics.

However, changes within the eyeball may occur, resulting in impaired vision. Objects that we once viewed with crystal clarity may become blurred or distorted. To better understand how vision may change, let's first examine the anatomy of the eye.

How the Eye Works

You may have heard the comparison between a camera and the human eye. Just as a camera takes in light and transforms it into an image on film, your eye does virtually the same thing, only the "film" is your retina and your brain "develops" the image. We see objects when light, which is reflected by the objects, passes through the eyeball lens and strikes the retina, at the back of the eye. Our brains then interpret the shapes, colors, and dimensions of the objects we see. A clearly focused object is the result of normal vision. However, just as an improper amount of light entering a camera lens will distort a photo, if light entering the eyeball does not strike the retina, the result may be distorted vision.

Anatomy of the Eye
Sclera and Cornea

The outer layer surrounding the eyeball is made up of two parts: the *sclera* and the *cornea*. The sclera—the white, opaque part of the eye—makes up the back five-sixths of the eye's outer layer and provides protection for the eyeball. The cornea, about the size of a dime and as thick as a credit card, makes up the remaining sixth of the eye's outer layer. It is the transparent dome, similar to the crystal of a wrist watch, at the front of the eyeball. The cornea provides most of the eye's focusing power, so small changes in its curvature can make an enormous difference in how clearly you see objects.

The Eyeball

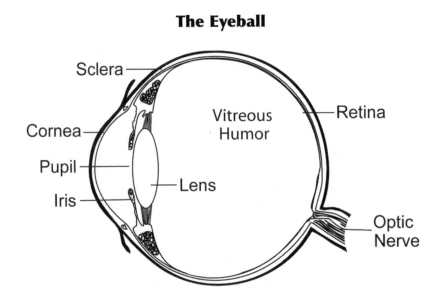

The *cornea* has three main layers. The *epithelium* is the thin outer protective layer of cells; it is made up of the same kind of tissue that covers most of your body, and is continually regenerating, or renewing itself. The *stroma* is the strong, fibrous layer that makes up 90 percent of the cornea's thickness and provides the cornea with its structure and shape. The *endothelium* is the single cell layer that lines the inside of the cornea and helps regulate the cornea's fluid content.

Iris

The *iris*, which determines one's eye color, is located behind the cornea. It is composed of connective tissue and smooth muscle fibers. The muscles of the iris control how much light passes through to the retina.

Pupil

The *pupil* appears as a black circle in the middle of the iris. The pupil can be likened to the aperture, or shutter, of a camera. When it is very bright, as on a sunny day, the iris muscles make the pupil constrict, or become small, so only a small amount of light will pass into the eye. In darkness the opposite happens, and the pupil dilates, or enlarges, to let in more light.

Normal Vision

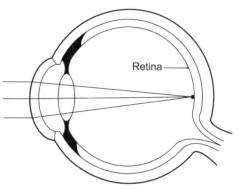

When one has normal vision, light rays enter through the lens and strike the retina, producing a focused image.

Lens

The *lens* is a circular structure located directly behind the pupil and held in place by slender, strong ligaments. Although most of the bending of light is accomplished by the cornea, the curved lens fine-tunes the angle of light passing through it, focusing the light onto the retina. When the ligaments tighten, the lens becomes flatter, or less convex, allowing you to see objects at a distance. When the ligaments relax, the elastic lens becomes rounder, or more convex, like a magnifying glass, so you can see objects that are close. This ability of the lens to refine the focus through flexing is called *accommodation*.

Vitreous Humor

The *vitreous humor* is the jellylike substance, about 99 percent water, that fills the space between the lens and the retina on the inner back wall of the eye. Light passes through the vitreous humor before striking the retina.

Retina

The *retina* is a complex layer of nerve tissue that lines the inside back wall of the eyeball. Similar to film in a camera, the retina "captures" the image through an electrochemical reaction to light. Electrical impulses are then transmitted through the *optic nerve* to the brain, which interprets, or "develops," the image.

Common Vision Problems

Your eye doctor may refer to your vision problem as your *refractive error*, or focusing problem. How well you see is determined, for the most part, by how accurately your eyes are able to bend, or *refract*, light. In a normal eye, the focus comes to a point on the retina. But sometimes this does not occur. The result? Various forms of vision impairment, or *aberrations*. Vision problems fall into one of two basic groups: *low-order aberrations* and *higher-order aberrations*.

Low-Order Aberrations
Myopia (Nearsightedness)

Also known as *nearsightedness*, *myopia* is a condition in which you can see nearby objects well, but objects at a distance appear blurred. This happens when light bouncing off a faraway image enters the eye through the cornea and comes to a point of focus too soon, before it reaches the retina. Myopia may be due to a cornea that has too much curvature, which causes the light to "overbend" and focus in front of the retina. Myopia also occurs when the eyeball is too long—the retinal wall is too far back for the combined focusing power of the cornea and lens.

Myopia

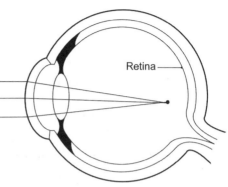

In myopia, or nearsightedness, light rays focus in front of the retina, causing distant objects to appear blurry.

Hyperopia

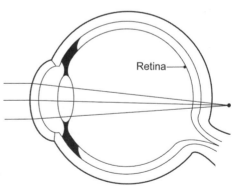

In hyperopia, or farsightedness, light rays focus behind the retina. Objects in the distance are seen more clearly than near objects.

Hyperopia (Farsightedness)

People with *hyperopia*, or *farsightedness*, see distant objects more clearly than nearby objects when they are young but may have difficulty with both as they get older. In hyperopia, the light rays coming into the cornea are not bent sharply enough and are focused behind, rather than on, the retina. The result is a blurred image. This usually happens in people whose eyeballs are too short from front to back or whose focusing muscles around the lens are too weak. Another cause of hyperopia, though rare, is a cornea that is not curved enough.

Because muscles are more elastic in youth, younger people who are mildly hyperopic can actually compensate for it by using the focusing muscles around the lens to fine-tune the focus by bending light more steeply. This action brings the point of focus forward toward the retina, allowing them to see more clearly. However, because the muscles weaken and the lens becomes less pliable as we age, these individuals eventually lose that ability and may no longer see well at a distance or close up. After age forty, they may be completely dependent on eyeglasses or contact lenses for both close and distant vision.

Astigmatism

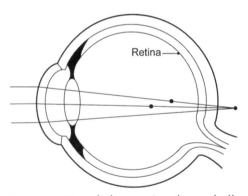

Retina→

In astigmatism, light entering the eyeball focuses on multiple areas rather than on the retina. Objects both far and near appear blurry

Astigmatism

Many individuals with myopia or hyperopia also have some degree of *astigmatism*. People with significant astigmatism experience blurred or distorted vision with all objects, whether near or far. Astigmatism means that your cornea, instead of being spherical like the side of a basketball, is slightly oval, shaped more like the side of a football. Your cornea is more curved in one direction than the other. As a result, light rays entering the eye from different points on the cornea's surface are bent irregularly and are focused at several different points, rather than meeting at just one focal point. Almost everyone has a small degree of astigmatism.

Presbyopia

Farsightedness is often confused with *presbyopia*, which literally means "old eyes." Presbyopia is the age-dependent need for reading glasses or bifocals. After age forty, and in most people by age forty-five, the ability to focus on an object close up, such as a restaurant menu, becomes more difficult. This happens to everyone. It is due to a loss of flexibility in the lens and a weakening in the muscles that enable the lens to flex and fine-tune the focus. Presbyopia typically continues to worsen until age sixty-five. When this occurs, people who already wear eyeglasses may need bifocals, and those who have never worn eyeglasses may require reading glasses.

Higher-Order Aberrations

Higher-order aberrations are focusing problems that are not correctable with glasses or contact lenses. Higher-order aberrations, which are a result of subtle irregularities in the focusing mechanism of the eye, cause a loss of crispness, clarity, and contrast. If you have significant higher-order aberrations, you may have trouble distinguishing between shades of gray. Higher-order aberrations may also affect one's night vision; people with these problems may see glare or halos around lights. Approximately 17 percent of visual errors are considered higher-order aberrations.

How Your Vision Is Measured

Most people who have had an eye exam that includes a test to measure *visual acuity*, clarity or sharpness of vision, recognize the simple notation 20/20 as meaning "normal vision." What do those numbers mean? Let's say your vision is 20/40. That means you can see at twenty feet what a person with normal vision can see at forty feet. Your measure of visual acuity is determined by using the *Snellen chart*, that familiar eye chart with progressively smaller letters on each line. Although it is considered an accurate vision test, its results are sometimes affected by such variables as squinting, guessing at the letters, and room light.

So, numbers such as 20/20 or 20/40 describe your visual acuity but do not measure your refractive error—how accurately your eye bends, or refracts, light. When an eye doctor measures your refractive error, what you end up with is your eyeglass prescription. Finding an eye doctor whose measurements are impeccable is crucial, not just for your eyeglass prescription but also, as you will learn later, for laser vision correction.

Understanding Your Eyeglass Prescription

Your eyeglass prescription is written in numbers. The type and degree of refractive error is quantified in units of measure called *diopters*. If you have ever wondered what those numbers mean, here is how to read and understand your prescription.

To arrive at your prescription, your doctor takes three measurements during the eye exam: sphere, cylinder, and axis. Your prescription for glasses may look something like this:

OD −1.25   —   —
OS −1.25 − .25 × 170

OD and OS refer to the right and left eyes, respectively. The first number next to OD or OS represents the *sphere*. The sphere measure tells the eye doctor where your eye focuses light: on the retina (normal vision), in front of the retina (myopia), or behind the retina (hyperopia). In other words, the sphere measure reveals whether you are nearsighted or farsighted. A negative diopter indicates myopia, or nearsightedness. A positive diopter indicates hyperopia, or farsightedness. The higher the number, the stronger the prescription. In the example above, the person has mild myopia (–1.25 diopters) in both eyes.

The number in the second column represents the *cylinder*. The cylinder measure indicates whether or not the patient has astigmatism. If the cylinder column is not blank, you have some degree of astigmatism. The larger the number, the more astigmatism you have. The example above reveals that this person has no astigmatism in the right eye, and a small amount (–.25 diopter) in the left eye.

If astigmatism is present, your eye doctor takes an *axis measurement*. The axis measure indicates where irregularity lies on the eyeball. In the prescription above, the astigmatism in the left eye is positioned at the 170-degree axis.

Nonsurgical Vision Correction Options

Eyeglasses

Eyeglasses have been around for hundreds of years. As early as the thirteenth century, inventors in China and Europe inserted magnifiers into frames, making the first prototype for our modern-day eyeglasses. Like the early versions, today's eyeglasses work like magnifying glasses that enhance the eye's ability to focus sharply, whether near or far. The amount of curvature in the spectacle lens determines how light bends before it reaches your cornea. Vision is corrected, depending on the angle of refraction, to compensate for your focusing error.

Eyeglasses have a number of advantages. They are usually affordable, are easy to maintain, and can be adapted for a number of different uses, such as reading, active sports, and driving. They also have disadvantages. Eyeglasses may restrict *peripheral vision*, the outer part of your field of vision; prove difficult in certain weather conditions, such as rain or snow; and make images appear smaller or larger than they really are. They may cause a number of visual aberrations, including halos around lights, and the lenses usually need to be replaced as your vision changes. Eyeglasses may interfere with certain occupations and recreational activities—swimming, for example. And some people just don't like the way they look in eyeglasses.

Contact Lenses

Contact lenses offer another option for correcting vision. Like eyeglasses, they make up the difference between the amount of refraction your eye can accomplish on its own and what is needed for sharp focus. Because they are extremely thin and are custom-shaped for your cornea, contact lenses float on the surface of your eye; they are held in place by natural suction and are constantly lubricated by the eye's own moisture.

Contact lenses have some advantages over eyeglasses. For example, contacts enable the wearer to have more natural vision (including better peripheral vision), cause little noticeable change in cosmetic appearance, and allow more freedom in recreational activities. On the other hand, contacts may require maintenance—continuous, frequent cleaning. Users must buy cleaning and storage solutions. The lenses may tear easily. They may be inconvenient for traveling, and also are easily lost. Contacts may be uncomfortable for patients with dry eyes or for those who live and work in polluted city air. They may cause visual aberrations (including halos and uneven vision) and always carry an increased risk of infection and possible corneal scarring. Individuals who live in higher altitudes may become intolerant of contact lenses over time because of the air's lower oxygen and humidity content.

The variety of contact lenses available today is dazzling. Costs for contacts vary widely, depending on the type you need.

Orthokeratology

This is a technique for treating myopia, or nearsightedness. *Orthokeratology* uses a series of rigid contact lenses that apply pressure to the cornea to flatten it. The effects are not permanent and require continued dependence on daily-wear maintenance lenses to retain the reshaping. Orthokeratology is generally only effective, even temporarily, for low levels of nearsightedness. The technique is expensive and high maintenance and requires continuous follow-up visits. Long-term effects can include permanently warped corneas. The risk of infection may also be greater than that from normal contact lens wear.

2

Laser Vision Correction: An Overview

People have understood the mechanics of eyesight for thousands of years. Writings and drawings on this subject go back as far as 2000 BC. And the quest to correct vision has never stopped. From the invention of eyeglasses hundreds of years ago to the fabrication of the first American contact lenses, the evolution of vision correction has indeed been astonishing. Now zoom ahead a few decades to the development of laser surgery, today one of the most popular methods of vision correction. The advent of computers and laser technology has made it possible to perform laser eye surgery to correct the shape of the cornea.

History of Vision Correction Surgery

Although many pioneering contributions led to the development of modern *refractive surgery*—that is, any surgical procedure to help the eye focus light correctly—a key breakthrough occurred in the middle of the last century. In 1949, Dr. José Barraquer of Bogotá, Colombia, developed the idea of lamellar corneal surgery ("lamellar" means "layered"). He discovered that lamellar surgery could reshape the cornea, enhancing the eye's ability to focus. To do so, Barraquer removed a disc of the front portion of the cornea with an instrument called a *microkeratome*. The instrument was affixed to the eye through use of a vacuum ring; then the *microkeratome* shaved a small amount of the cornea at a predetermined depth. Dr. Barraquer froze the disc and then ground it into a new shape with a small lathe. He placed the newly shaped disc back on the cornea. The procedure of carving the cornea was called keratomileusis.

Two important refinements followed. In 1985, Dr. Casimir Swinger developed a method of reshaping the disc without freezing it (*nonfreeze keratomileusis*). Then, in 1987, Dr. Luis Ruiz, a protégé of Barraquer, used an automated microkeratome to reshape the cornea directly on the eye. This procedure, *automated lamellar keratoplasty* (ALK), was used to correct high levels of myopia and hyperopia. It is important to note that patients who have undergone these two procedures, precursors to today's laser vision correction, have not experienced long-term complications from the corneal reshaping.

The Arrival of the Excimer Laser

The *excimer laser* was first used on human eyes in the late 1980s. The laser technology marked a significant advancement in the science of vision correction; the excimer laser uses a cool ultraviolet beam of light to vaporize tissue—that is, break up the molecules—with exacting precision and without harming adjacent tissue. Each pulse of the excimer laser removes a mere 1/100,000 inch of tissue.

Photorefractive Keratectomy (PRK)

The procedure that originally made wide use of the excimer laser was *photorefractive keratectomy* (PRK), first performed in 1987. Instead of using a microkeratome to remove the corneal disc, PRK uses the laser to accurately sculpt the cornea one microscopic layer at a time. PRK has seen vast improvements since those early days.

PRK sculpts the cornea by first removing the epithelium, the outer protective layer of the cornea. The laser works its way down into the stroma, or structural part of the cornea, where the real reshaping takes place. The epithelium then grows back over the next forty-eight to seventy-two hours. PRK presents some inconveniences. First, PRK can leave your eye sore for twenty-four to forty-eight hours after surgery while the eye heals. Second, the corneal surface, left exposed, results in blurred vision for almost a week. (See chapter 9 on PRK.)

LASIK

In 1990, researchers conceived of ways to avoid these side effects associated with PRK; they developed a new procedure called LASIK, a type of refractive surgery, in which a laser is used to reshape the cornea, improving vision. LASIK is an acronym for *laser-assisted in situ keratomileusis*. The component words of LASIK are defined as:

LASer-assisted—performed with the excimer laser.

In situ—the laser sculpting is performed on the cornea after a flap of corneal tissue has been lifted.

Keratomileusis—a process of carving the cornea to reshape it.

During a LASIK procedure, the outermost layers of the cornea are peeled back, using a thin blade or laser called a microkeratome. This creates an extremely thin flap, which, like a hinged lid, is gently lifted back, exposing the corneal tissue beneath. The cornea is then precisely sculpted by the excimer laser into a new shape to correct the vision. The flap is set back in place. The flap is held in position by the eye's natural suction.

Clinical trials on LASIK began in the United States in 1991. A broad series of clinical investigations culminated in its approval by

Layers of the Cornea

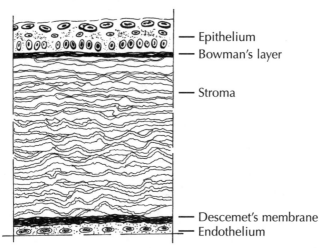

— Epithelium
— Bowman's layer
— Stroma
— Descemet's membrane
— Endothelium

The cornea, about as thick as a credit card, is made up of many layers. When LASIK is performed, surgeons reshape the stroma layer, changing the way light bends as it enters the eye.

the FDA in 1999.

How LASIK Corrects the Eye's Focus

How can a laser beam correct vision? The excimer laser is uniquely suited to the task of refractive corneal surgery because it ablates, or vaporizes, tissue by breaking apart the molecules without creating damaging heat. The unparalleled precision of the excimer laser makes it the ultimate reshaping tool. The laser is so precise that it would take 600 pulses to break through one strand of human hair. This precision allows the surgeon to sculpt the exposed corneal bed, gently and precisely, into a more desirable shape that allows rays of light to focus properly on the retina. The result is improved vision.

LASIK and Myopic Correction

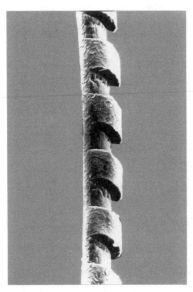

This human hair, which has been ablated by an excimer laser, shows the precision with which the laser works. (*Photo courtesy of Advanced Medical Optics.*)

As explained earlier, patients who are nearsighted have corneas with too much curvature in proportion to the length of their eyes. Once the corneal flap is made and lifted back, the excimer laser reshapes the underlying stroma to achieve a flatter cornea. The surgeon's careful, precise measurements, programmed into the computer, guide the excimer laser. When the reshaping is complete, the flap is replaced. The result is that light rays coming through the cornea now come to a point of focus on the retina, rather than in front of it.

LASIK and Hyperopic Correction

Farsighted patients, on the other hand, have corneas that are proportionately too flat for the length of their eyes. The excimer laser is programmed to remove tissue from just the periphery of the stroma, leaving the middle untouched; this creates more of a domed shape. The increased curvature of the cornea will allow light rays to focus on the retina, rather than behind it.

LASIK and Astigmatism

To treat astigmatism, the excimer laser removes tissue in a somewhat oval fashion, adjusting the shape of the cornea in one direction more than the other. The goal is to produce a symmetrical surface so that light rays passing through the cornea at various places will meet at a single point of focus on the retina.

LASIK: State of the Art

No LASIK surgeon can promise 20/20 vision without the use of corrective eyeglasses or contact lenses. However, more than 99 percent of typical myopic patients after LASIK can see well enough to legally drive without glasses, usually by the morning after surgery. With today's technological advances, the typical patient has a greater than 95 percent chance of achieving 20/20 vision. (See more on wavefront technology in chapter 5.)

3

Contemplating Laser Eye Surgery

If you have worn eyeglasses or contacts most of your life, the possibility of having good eyesight without them may have seemed remote. But today high success rates with LASIK and PRK are inspiring more people to seriously contemplate laser eye surgery. A good way to get started is to address these two questions: Am I a good candidate for LASIK, and how do I find the best surgeon?

Am I a Good Candidate for LASIK?

Whether LASIK is the best option for you will ultimately depend on the judgment of your eye surgeon, who will make that determination during a preoperative evaluation. However, good candidates for LASIK have some basic conditions in common.

Ideal Age

A good candidate is at least eighteen years old, because the vision of people younger than eighteen years often continues to change. Myopia may continue to increase in some patients until their mid- to late twenties.

Stable Prescription

No matter what your age, to be considered a good candidate for LASIK, your vision prescription should be stable. In practical terms, your prescription is stable if your glasses or contacts are at least a year old and you still see well with them.

Treatable Eyesight Parameters

A good candidate for LASIK has an eyeglass prescription that falls within certain parameters. If you are nearsighted, you may have myopia of up to −12.00 diopters. If you are farsighted, your hyperopia may be up to +6.00 diopters. Your level of astigmatism may be as high as 6.00 diopters. These are normal parameters, but they can vary from patient to patient and from doctor to doctor.

Surgically Ideal Eyes

You will not know until the preoperative examination whether your eyes meet the standards required for LASIK. These would include:

- A cornea of the right thickness (not too thin)
- A cornea that is structurally normal (not irregularly shaped)
- Generally healthy eyes (no eye diseases or injuries that could interfere with the outcome)

Conditions That May Prevent Surgery

Any number of factors could make you a poor candidate for LASIK. Some patients fear their eyesight is too poor, yet later discover, after meeting with their eye doctor, that it falls within treatable parameters that yield successful outcomes. So, do not assume you are a poor candidate until you have consulted with your eye doctor and he or she confirms it.

Some people aren't good candidates for LASIK. When I recommend against the surgery, my concern is that these patients will go somewhere else and have the surgery done when they shouldn't.

Dr. Robert Maloney

Severe Refractive Error

If your refractive error is so severe that it falls outside normal treatable parameters, you may not be a candidate for LASIK. To correct extreme nearsightedness or farsightedness requires too much deep sculpting and corneal reshaping. Other vision correction procedures, such as the implantable contact lens (see appendix) may be preferable. But to be certain, get your eye doctor's opinion.

Other Health Conditions

You may be a poor candidate for LASIK if you have any of the following conditions:

- *Thin cornea.* LASIK will not weaken a normal cornea, but if your cornea is unusually thin, LASIK could weaken it, causing distortion in your vision. If you have a thin cornea, PRK may be a better option for you, because it won't weaken a thin cornea. (See chapter 9, PRK.)

- *Abnormally structured cornea.* This condition is not treatable with LASIK.

- *Pregnancy.* Vision can be unstable during pregnancy, especially during the third trimester. As a result, the measured refraction may be inaccurate. On the other hand, if a woman is early in her pregnancy and her vision hasn't changed, it may be possible in special cases to do LASIK.

- *Cataract.* Cataract is a clouding of the lens within the eye that causes blurry vision. If you have a cataract, LASIK can accentuate the blurring of vision caused by the cataract.

- *Corneal dystrophies.* These are inherited conditions in which one or more parts of the cornea lose normal clarity due to a buildup of cloudy material.

- *A history of ocular herpetic keratitis.* The same herpes virus that causes cold sores on the lips can cause recurring infection in the eye, resulting in scarring and blurred vision. This is not a sexually transmitted disease.

- *Diabetic retinopathy.* This is a potentially blinding complication of diabetes that damages the eye's retina. Patients with diabetes who have normal corneal sensation and do not have retinopathy are usually candidates for LASIK, however.

- *Severe dry eye.* Patients with severe dry eye can have healing problems after LASIK. On the other hand, mild to moderate dry eye that is treated before surgery does not cause healing problems, so this condition does not automatically mean LASIK is not an option.

Although the conditions listed above are generally contraindications to LASIK, none are absolute contraindications. If you have one of these conditions, consultation with an experienced LASIK surgeon will help you determine whether LASIK is still a possibility for you.

Unrealistic Expectations

If you have unrealistic expectations, you may be disappointed with the outcome of laser eye surgery. As a patient, you are responsible for understanding exactly what the procedure can and cannot do. For example, you might still need eyeglasses for performing certain activities, such as viewing a subtitled film or driving at night. It is best to think of LASIK as reducing your dependence on eyeglasses and contact lenses and improving your natural vision.

Issues to Discuss with Your Doctor

The following factors represent areas of controversy in terms of whether a patient is a good candidate for LASIK. Some eye doctors recommend avoiding LASIK surgery, while others believe that decisions need to be made on a case-by-case basis. If you have any of these conditions, discuss them with your eye surgeon.

- *Unusually large pupils.* One of the potential side effects of LASIK is glare or seeing halos around lights at night. If you have unusually large pupils, more light enters your eyes at night. Some doctors believe that this extra light causes more glare and halos. A number of major studies have now shown that this is not the case, that there is little if any correlation between pupil size and night vision. More and more doctors are coming to agree with us that pupil size is relatively unimportant to your candidacy for LASIK.

- *Nursing mothers.* Some doctors are concerned that vision may change while a mother is nursing. This is not our experience. If more than two months have passed since delivery, you are a candidate for LASIK. However, if you are nursing and do have the surgery, we recommend you don't take any oral sedatives, like Valium, that your doctor routinely offers, because they will get into your breast milk.

- *Pacemakers.* Some pacemakers that are more than twenty years old can be affected by electromagnetic fields emitted by equipment like the excimer laser. Patients with older pacemakers can still have LASIK, but they may require that a technician be present to oversee the pacemaker. Newer pacemaker models are unaffected by the laser.

- *Autoimmune diseases.* These diseases are caused by an abnormal attack by your immune system on the natural, healthy cells of your body. Certain autoimmune diseases, such as rheumatoid arthritis, are rarely associated with corneal melting, or dissolving, in patients who have eye surgery. These conditions can also cause severe dry eye. In general, we find that if you have an autoimmune disease but are under age sixty-five and don't have severe dryness, you may be a candidate for LASIK.

- *The use of certain prescription medicines.* Some doctors believe that certain prescription medicines impair healing. These prescription drugs include Accutane, used to treat severe acne; amiodarone, prescribed to treat irregular heartbeat; and oral steroids, often used by individuals with severe allergies, with asthma, or with inflammatory diseases such as arthritis and lupus. Tell your eye doctor about any prescription and over-the-counter medications you are taking.

Finding the Right LASIK Surgeon

If you are a candidate for LASIK, your next step will be the most important one: finding the right physician to perform the procedure. You will need an *ophthalmologist* to perform your LASIK surgery. An ophthalmologist is a licensed medical doctor who has a minimum of four years of additional training after medical school. This advanced training usually involves a one-year internship in internal medicine or general surgery,

The most important thing is that a patient's expectations be met. The only way for a doctor to do that is to spend time with a patient and learn about why he or she wants the procedure and what the patient's goals are.

Dr. Ernest Kornmehl

followed by three or four years in an ophthalmology residency. A select group of ophthalmologists complete an additional year or two of fellowship training in corneal or refractive surgery. Following are some suggestions to help you identify the most qualified surgeons.

Ask Other Patients

If you know people who have had the LASIK procedure, ask them who their surgeon was and how they felt about their overall experience. Were they happy with the outcome? Did they have confidence in their surgeon? Was the surgeon compassionate, and did he or she take time to answer questions before and after the procedure? Was the support staff helpful? Personal experiences are powerful indicators of the quality of care.

Ask Your Eye Doctor

An eye care practitioner whom you trust and respect is another good source of referrals. Because referring patients is a routine and important part of their professional practice, these physicians will almost always be able to recommend a nearby LASIK surgeon with a sound reputation.

Contact Ophthalmic Boards and Medical Associations

Some medical organizations, such as the American Board of Ophthalmology, provide information about physicians free of charge to consumers. Ask for names of ophthalmologists who specialize in corneal and refractive surgery who have been certified by the board. The American Academy of Ophthalmology also has a Web site, www.aao.org, where you may search for member eye doctors by city, state, and specialty (refractive surgery). The site lists doctors' practice focus, current professional activity, educational history and degrees, residency, fellowships, teaching positions, board certification, contact information, and often a Web site address. More information on how to contact this organization is listed in the resource section in the back of this book.

The International Society of Refractive Surgery also maintains a list of member surgeons on its Web site, www.isrs.org. This list is less comprehensive than the American Academy of Ophthalmology list for US surgeons but is a better list for finding surgeons outside the United States. Note that membership in this and other organizations does not necessarily mean the surgeon is board certified.

Check your local library for the four-volume *Official ABMS Directory of Board Certified Medical Specialists.* This publication lists by region refractive surgeons who have been certified by the American Board of Ophthalmology. To verify whether a specific eye doctor is board certified, you can also call ABMS at 866-ASK-ABMS (275-2267), or go on the ABMS Web site at www.abms.org.

Using the Internet

If you like doing consumer research on the Internet, you will find much information about LASIK online. Keep in mind, however, that the Internet is an unsupervised and largely unregulated medium. Much of the information about LASIK on the Internet is either inaccurate or incomplete.

> The three most important qualities in a surgeon are: obsessive attention to detail, statistical sophistication in analyzing surgery results, and having a lot of experience.
>
> Dr. Robert Maloney

You may also find commercial directories, both online and elsewhere, that list surgeons who perform LASIK. Surgeons pay to be included in these listings much like the yellow pages, so the sites are of limited use. Most of them do not check a surgeon's credentials, so be sure to research the doctors' credentials thoroughly.

Questions to Ask Your Surgeon

Once you have the names of refractive surgeons, the next step is to find out more about their credentials, reputation, and practice. Don't be shy about asking penetrating questions. LASIK surgeons understand that patients have many questions about them and about the procedure, and they should be prepared to answer the questions for you. When you find a doctor with promising credentials, call the office and ask to speak with the LASIK coordinator or a staff member who can answer your questions.

What Are the Surgeon's Credentials?

Consider only surgeons who are board certified. What does this mean? In addition to the medical education, internship, and residency program mentioned earlier, ophthalmologists must pass a series of exams given by the National Board of Medical Examiners; they must also pass two additional examinations administered by the American Board of Ophthalmology. After passing these final exams, physicians are certified by the American Board of Ophthalmology. About 90 percent of ophthalmologists eventually pass these exams, so the designation "board-certified" does not help you separate outstanding surgeons from merely good ones. However, lack of board certification is a warning sign—it means the doctor is in the bottom 10 percent of ophthalmologists in knowledge of the field.

Some ophthalmologists are *fellowship-trained* cornea or refractive surgeons. This means they have been offered one or two years of extra training in diseases and surgery of the cornea under the supervision of leading physicians in the field. Fellowship-trained surgeons will likely have a lower incidence of complications, because they can diagnose subtle findings prior to surgery.

How Many LASIK Procedures Has the Surgeon Performed?

Be specific in asking about a physician's experience with LASIK, because other laser procedures require skills different from those required for LASIK. Because there is a learning curve, surgeons should have performed a minimum of 1,000 LASIK procedures; research shows that the complication rate for surgeons is reduced even further after they have performed 3,000 procedures.

It generally takes that many LASIK procedures before a surgeon's *nomogram* is reasonably well developed. The nomogram refers to the formula the surgeon enters into the excimer laser computer for each procedure. Even though excimer lasers come from the manufacturer with recommended settings to correct the various refractive errors, the surgeon fine-tunes and customizes these settings with the nomogram. Based on a series of measurements the surgeon takes during the preoperative exam, the nomogram includes factors such as the degree of refractive error and the patient's age. It also takes into consideration the surgeon's own technique and the type of laser he or she will use. A well-developed and artful nomogram allows the surgeon to more accurately program the laser for each patient, increasing the likelihood of perfect vision.

How Many Procedures Has the Surgeon Performed on Patients with Your Refractive Error?

Perhaps as important as the total number of LASIK procedures a surgeon has completed is the number he or she has performed on patients with the same refractive error as yours, using the same laser equipment. The surgeon should have completed 100 or more such procedures. Even an experienced surgeon could have difficulty with certain less common refractive errors. And new equipment takes some

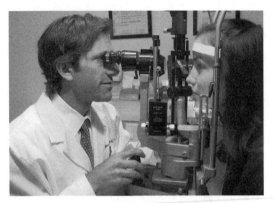

As part of the screening for a LASIK procedure, Dr. Jonathan Davidorf, ophthalmologist, performs a microscopic exam of a patient's corneas, checking for possible abnormalities.

getting used to as well. Additionally, the surgeon should have experience with patients of your age and race—relevant because the surgical techniques needed to correct refractive errors in these groups may differ slightly.

Ask to Speak with Former Patients

Ask a prospective surgeon for the names of two or three patients you can contact who had a refractive error similar to yours. This is not an unusual request. When you speak with them, ask how they felt about the surgeon, the staff, and the quality of their LASIK experience.

How Does the Surgeon Track LASIK Procedure Outcomes?

The surgeon's response to this question will reveal much. If the surgeon has readily available statistics in the form of charts and graphs, he or she is most likely *benchmarking*, or tracking, LASIK outcomes. In addition, if the surgeon presents his or her data to other surgeons at well-respected national or international conferences, or publishes in professional journals, you can be confident that he or she is tracking outcomes.

Benchmarking is very important, because it indicates the surgeon is concerned about achieving the best possible results over time. There is no mandatory central reporting database for tracking LASIK outcomes, unless a surgeon is participating in a sanctioned clinical trial. Therefore, a surgeon's doing so voluntarily indicates high personal standards of professionalism and performance.

It is important in tracking data that your surgeon has performed a statistically significant number of procedures. With data from 3,000 or more procedures, your surgeon would be able to predict outcomes fairly accurately.

What Are the Surgeon's Success and Complication Rates?

The surgeon should be able to give you the percentage of LASIK patients whose procedures result in 20/20 vision or better. It's normal for more than 80 percent of LASIK patients to achieve this level of vision. In fact, with wavefront-guided treatment, which uses newer diagnostic technology, most patients in a top practice today have a 95 percent chance of achieving 20/20 vision. (See more details on wavefront in chapter 5.) With data based on 1,000 or more procedures, your surgeon should be able to tell your chances of achieving a good result with LASIK and whether you will need an enhancement procedure. Ask what percentage of LASIK patients report significant complications. Less than 1 percent is acceptable. Keep in mind that most complications, if they do occur, can be managed by an experienced surgeon.

Has the Surgeon Participated in Research Activities, Lecturing, or Writing?

Doctors who have researched and written articles for peer-reviewed journals, been speakers at medical conferences, and/or published books are usually well respected among their peers. This is an indication of a physician's experience and competence. This level of professional involvement, above and beyond his or her ophthalmology practice, shows the doctor's mastery of, motivation in, and passion for the field.

Has the Surgeon Ever Participated in an FDA Clinical Trial?

The U.S. Food and Drug Administration (FDA) authorizes some ophthalmologists to participate as principal investigators in *clinical trials* sponsored by laser manufacturers. A clinical trial is a research study, conducted with patients, that is designed to evaluate the safety and effectiveness of a new procedure or device. Typically, FDA-authorized ophthalmologists are chosen because of their demonstrated skill and ability and their complete understanding of laser vision correction and the laser being used. These surgeons are subject to detailed analysis and reporting and are willing to endure extreme scrutiny.

Note that an ophthalmologist may have never been asked to participate in a clinical trial, yet may be very competent to perform LASIK. Still, if you've found a surgeon who has participated in a clinical trial, you're more likely to have found one of the best.

Has the Doctor Ever Been Sued for Malpractice?

Even the best surgeon may have had a malpractice suit brought against him or her, so be careful about passing judgment based on what might have been a frivolous lawsuit. The typical vision correction surgeon is sued roughly once for every 3000 surgeries performed. Statistics indicate that about 80 percent of these suits are either frivolous or without merit. If the doctor has been sued more frequently than this, or has multiple simultaneous lawsuits, you should ask for an explanation. If you are embarrassed to ask about malpractice suits against the doctor, there are alternative ways to obtain this information.

One organization, the Association of State Medical Board Executive Directors, is a group of participating state licensing authorities that provides malpractice and disciplinary action information about specific doctors. The association's information is free and available at its Web site, www.docboard.org. However, not every state in the nation participates.

The Federation of State Medical Boards is another organization that collects and disseminates information about doctors' malpractice histories. It takes five to seven days to get an answer to a request. Contact the organization at its Web site, www.fsmb.org, or write to it at the address listed in the resource section.

Has the Doctor Been Sanctioned by the State Medical Board?

All doctors must be licensed by the state medical board in any state in which they practice. Medical boards will discipline doctors for significant misbehavior, including gross or repeated acts of negligence. Contact your state medical board for information on the doctor you are considering. Many state medical boards now publish disciplinary actions against surgeons online.

How Many Patients Does the Surgeon Turn Away?

A conscientious surgeon will turn away about 10 percent of the patients he or she evaluates during the preoperative examination. Be wary of a doctor who rarely advises a patient against the procedure. Many factors can make a patient a poor candidate for LASIK. No doctor with high ethical standards will perform laser surgery on your eyes if you are not a good candidate.

Will the Doctor Be Personally Involved in Evaluating Me for Surgery?

Avoid the "shopping mall" approach to surgery, where patients are shuffled through to the surgical suite without first having met with the surgeon. Most doctors have knowledgeable and compassionate staff to help perform tests and answer questions. However, it is also important to meet the surgeon and receive his or her personal evaluation before you decide to have the surgery.

Some patients choose to see their regular eye doctor for their preoperative and postoperative care. If you plan to do this, be sure your surgeon is comfortable working with your primary eye doctor. While the majority of people have an uncomplicated postoperative course, you want to make sure your care provider will be able to recognize complications if they arise and can either treat you or refer you for treatment before more serious, long-term repercussions occur.

What Type of Laser Does the Surgeon Use?

Make sure your doctor uses a newest-generation excimer laser that is capable of performing wavefront-guided treatment. Laser technology has improved dramatically over past years. State-of-the-art lasers now have eye tracking, which further improves the safety of the procedure. If your eye moves accidentally during the treatment, the laser automatically tracks, or follows, it. Make sure your surgeon uses an eye-tracking laser. State-of-the-art lasers enable surgeons to treat larger areas, minimizing the risk of nighttime glare.

The FDA Web site, www.fda.gov, also has links to laser manufacturers' Web sites, where some maintain lists of doctors certified to use their machines. If your doctor is not listed, you may wish to contact the laser manufacturer directly. Verify that the doctor has been certified by the laser company to operate a particular machine, which means he or she took a required training course.

How Much Does LASIK Cost?

Cost should not be the main factor in choosing a LASIK surgeon. First and foremost, seek out a surgeon who has a good reputation in the medical community and plenty of experience. If you are swayed by low cost, this may signal trouble for you down the road. Find the best-qualified surgeon with high medical standards for patient care, compassionate staff to tend to your needs, comprehensive postoperative care, enhancement procedures if necessary, and availability if any problems or complications crop up after surgery.

The cost of LASIK varies from surgeon to surgeon. Generally, high-quality, wavefront-guided LASIK runs between $2,200 and $3,000 per eye. Be sure to ask whether the quoted per-eye cost includes preoperative and postoperative care, as well as enhancement procedures. Many practices can help you arrange low-interest or no-interest financing, which makes high-quality surgery affordable for almost everyone.

Making the Decision

Sometimes, no matter how much information you have gathered, the decision to choose one surgeon over another comes down to intuition. Personal chemistry is important. Choose someone with whom you feel comfortable—someone who is easy to talk to, friendly, and professional. Naturally, you also want a surgeon who listens to your questions, answers them completely, and asks you questions as well. A good doctor patient relationship is important in devising a treatment plan that best suits your needs. Likewise, the surgeon's support staff should be highly trained, competent, and caring. These are the people who will help support you through the LASIK procedure.

Once you feel comfortable with your decision—after you've carefully researched surgeons in your area—you're probably ready to schedule your initial consultation.

4

Your Consultation

Your consultation is your opportunity to become fully informed about LASIK and decide whether or not the procedure is right for you. You will learn about the strengths and limitations of the procedure as it applies to your eyes. Often a comprehensive examination of your eyes will be done at the initial visit to ensure that you are a good candidate. At some point in the process, you should get to know the surgeon and have the opportunity to ask as many questions as necessary in order to feel safe and comfortable undergoing LASIK. Many patients prefer to invite a friend, their spouse, or another family member to sit in on the meeting with the surgeon. He or she may help you remember questions to ask or may help you recall information later.

Before surgery, the surgeon should take the opportunity to get to know you, gain an understanding of your expectations, and do an examination of your eyes. After a comprehensive examination of your eyes, the surgeon should be able to tell whether you are a good candidate for LASIK and what your outcome will likely be.

Unfortunately, some LASIK centers use a high-pressure sales approach, almost like selling used cars. There is some chance that these centers may recommend LASIK even if you are not a good candidate. We recommend that if you feel you are getting a sales job, you should leave and go elsewhere. LASIK is fundamentally a medical procedure and should be treated as such.

The Initial Appointment

The preoperative consultation usually takes about an hour and a half. When you call to make an appointment, you will be asked about the type of contact lenses you wear, if any. You'll also be given instructions about your contacts in preparation for the consultation.

- If you wear soft spherical contact lenses, you should stop wearing them forty eight hours to one week before your consultation.

- If you wear soft toric contact lenses, you should also stop wearing them seventy-two hours to two weeks before your consultation, depending on surgeon preference. Toric lenses are soft lenses designed for astigmatism. They are slightly oval-shaped and are weighted so they will not rotate on the eye.

- If you wear hard contact lenses or rigid gas permeable (RGP) lenses, you may need to stop wearing them for several weeks before your consultation. RGP lenses are made of a porous substance that permits oxygen to permeate the lenses so the eyes can "breathe."

Why discontinue wearing contact lenses prior to the eye exam? Contact lenses can alter the shape of your cornea for up to several weeks after you have stopped wearing them, depending on the type of lens. For the surgeon to take accurate measurements, the cornea must assume its natural shape. Your surgeon may need to repeat these measurements after your initial consultation and before surgery to make sure the shape of your cornea has stabilized. If you wear your contacts to the consultation appointment, the surgeon can usually tell you whether you are a candidate, but he or she can't take accurate measurements of your eyes until after you discontinue lens wear.

Your Medical and Vision History

When you meet with your surgeon for the first time, he or she will want to get a sense of your overall health and the health of your eyes. It is important for your surgeon to know everything about your medical history. Some systemic diseases—like rheumatoid arthritis and lupus—certain healing disorders, diabetes, and a current or planned pregnancy demand special consideration when it comes to laser vision correction.

Also tell your surgeon about any ongoing changes or problems you have had with your vision. For example, if you have a significant cataract, you should not undergo LASIK vision correction. Symptoms of cataract include glare from lamps or very bright light, frequent changes in your eyeglass prescription, and cloudy or blurred vision.

Be sure to tell your surgeon about any problems you've had with contact lenses, or any other eye-related discomfort you have been having. For example, patients often turn to laser eye surgery when their contacts have become too uncomfortable to wear because of dry eyes.

The Comprehensive Examination

The next part of the preoperative evaluation involves a series of eye tests and examinations that provide the necessary data before a LASIK procedure. These may be conducted at your surgeon's office or by your regular eye doctor.

In either case, the physician will measure your refractive error and determine which of your eyes is dominant. Next, he or she will measure your cornea with a *corneal topographer*, an instrument that uses computerized analysis to arrive at an extremely accurate three-dimensional map of your cornea. This test will reveal whether you have a structurally abnormal cornea, which could disqualify you as a candidate for LASIK.

The thickness of your cornea will be measured with a *pachymeter*. Because a certain amount of tissue will be surgically removed, or ablated, during the LASIK procedure, your cornea must be thick enough for the remaining tissue to retain its structure and shape. If your cornea is too thin, you would not be a good LASIK candidate.

The surgeon will examine your eyes with a special microscope called a *slit lamp*. This allows examination of the cornea in microscopic detail. The doctor will be checking for abnormalities that could be symptomatic of eye disease.

The *intraocular pressure* of your eyes will be measured with a *tonometer*. This tests the pressure exerted by the fluid (aqueous humor) within the eyeball that gives it a round, firm shape. Increased pressure could be an indication of glaucoma.

Next, drops may be put in your eyes. These drops temporarily relax focusing muscles, dilating the pupil. The doctor may measure your refractive error again and will examine the back of the eye, including the retina and the optic nerve. In nearsighted patients, these dilating eyedrops will not affect distance vision, which is needed for driving, but will blur near vision for about four to six hours. Both near and distance vision may be affected in farsighted patients.

Common Questions about LASIK

LASIK surgeons are accustomed to having patients ask questions. Part of the physician's role is to educate you as thoroughly as possible.

Many LASIK centers offer written material designed to address your questions. Other LASIK centers show short videos that explain the procedure in detail. However, if you still have questions, or just want to discuss any reservations or fears, the consultation is the best time to do it.

Is LASIK Painful?

No. Before the procedure begins, your eye is numbed with eyedrops. You may feel a slight sensation of pressure as the corneal flap is being made, but the procedure should not hurt at all. After the surgery, any discomfort you experience will last only a few hours. Sleep and lubricating eyedrops, as well as acetaminophen or ibuprofen, are usually enough to take care of any discomfort.

> *Some patients want to know about the procedure down to every last detail, while others don't wish to discuss it. Nonetheless, every patient needs to be informed.*
>
> *Dr. Jonathan Davidorf*

How Long Does the LASIK Procedure Take?

Most patients are pleasantly surprised at how quickly LASIK is performed. Expect an experienced surgeon to complete the procedure in five to ten minutes per eye.

How Long Will It Take for My Eyes to Heal?

The healing process is remarkably fast, with few associated side effects. Most postoperative discomfort and visual side effects are quite minor. You may notice a burning sensation and may experience watery eyes in one or both eyes for a few hours after surgery, but usually by the very next day, you should not have any significant eye discomfort. The most common discomfort that sometimes persists is dry eye. This occurs because the nerves in the cornea are temporarily altered when the corneal flap is made during the procedure.

Symptoms related to post-LASIK dry eye are usually minor, can be alleviated with lubricating eyedrops, and generally disappear within two to six months. In terms of visual acuity, most patients notice good vision the day after surgery. Visual clarity and crispness after LASIK tends to improve for two to six months and then stabilizes.

What Results Can I Expect?

Results vary. Finding a skilled and experienced surgeon maximizes your chances for the best possible outcome. However, with higher degrees of myopia, hyperopia, and astigmatism, results are less predictable and enhancement procedures are more common.

How Long Will the Correction Last?

Once your eye has stabilized, usually in two to three months, your correction is permanent. If you eventually need eyeglasses for reading after that, it would be the result of the normal aging process.

What about Risks and Complications?

It is not unusual for people considering LASIK to experience fear, nervousness, and uncertainty at first. Most patients feel a lot better about the procedure once they become fully informed. Knowing the statistical improbability of a serious complication goes a long way toward relieving your fears.

Your doctor should inform you about the risks and potential complications associated with LASIK, ranging from very minor, short-term discomfort to serious complications, which are rare. He or she should also explain what you can do to avoid some of these risks. Fortunately, the incidence of serious complications is low in the hands of a competent surgeon. More details about risks and possible complications appear in chapter 8.

Will I Be Able to Drive Immediately after LASIK?

State departments of motor vehicles typically grant unrestricted driving privileges to people with 20/40 or better vision. More than 90 percent of all patients who undergo LASIK have this level of vision or better the day after surgery.

When Can I Go Back to Work?

Most patients can return to work the day after their LASIK procedure. If you work in a very dusty environment, such as a construction site, wait a couple of days before going back to work.

Although most patients can function normally at work the day after surgery, your vision may still be somewhat blurry and your eyes may be occasionally irritated, so we recommend that you not schedule any critical appointments or meetings for that day.

Will I Need Enhancement Surgery?

About 10 percent of LASIK patients require *enhancement procedures*. For example, if an eye is undercorrected or overcorrected with LASIK, you can undergo an enhancement procedure. Even in the hands of the most skilled surgeon, each person's tissue responds differently to the excimer laser, both during the surgery and while healing. If you do need an enhancement procedure, you must wait for your eye must stabilize, which usually takes three to six months after the original surgery.

When an enhancement procedure is performed, the corneal flap will not need to be re-created. Instead, the surgeon, using a specialized instrument, gently lifts the preexisting flap and performs the additional laser treatment. Recovery time is similar to that of the original procedure. You may or may not be charged an additional fee for such enhancement surgery. Keep in mind that enhancement procedures can also be performed years later if your eyesight changes over time.

If I Have Dry Eyes, Will It Affect My LASIK Surgery?

Many patients consider LASIK because they have dry eyes and cannot wear contact lenses. If you have significant dryness, your doctor may recommend treatment before surgery. Tear supplements and *punctum plugs* (tiny silicone plugs placed in the tear drainage openings of your eyelid) should keep your eyes moist.

After LASIK, your eyes may feel drier. This condition typically improves from one week to six months after surgery. Symptoms of dry eye can be particularly noticeable if you use a computer frequently, read for long periods of time, or drive extended distances. For many patients, it is useful to use lubricating eyedrops often, especially for the first few weeks after surgery.

If you have external eye diseases such as *meibomitis* (inflammation of the inner lid) or *blepharitis* (debris at the base of the eyelashes), your doctor may want to treat these conditions prior to a laser vision correction procedure.

If I've Had Previous Eye Surgery, Am I Still a Candidate for LASIK?

Patients who have had certain types of eye surgery are sometimes candidates for LASIK as a second procedure to improve their vision. However, these are often more difficult surgeries and have less predictable results.

For example, LASIK has been used following an older form of refractive surgery, *radial keratotomy (RK)*. With RK, the cornea is flattened by making small, spokelike incisions around its periphery to correct myopia and astigmatism. LASIK following RK can succeed as long as the patient's vision is relatively stable and there is no significant corneal scarring or epithelial debris in the incisions.

Patients who have had a *corneal transplant* can have a LASIK procedure to enhance results. This is especially effective for those who developed a high degree of astigmatism caused by the surgery. A clear corneal transplant will allow good vision only if it has a relatively round surface. Laser vision correction can smooth out astigmatic curves in the cornea.

If I Have Thin Corneas, Am I Still a Candidate for LASIK?

You may be if you have a mild refractive error. If your cornea is thin, removing the amount of tissue necessary to correct your vision may weaken your cornea. A careful surgeon will calculate the amount of tissue removed to ensure your cornea is not weakened. If too much tissue will be removed, the surgeon will recommend PRK or an implantable contact lens instead.

> *Follow-up care is important, too. I encourage patients to ask a lot of questions about the quality of follow-up care they'll receive after a LASIK procedure.*
>
> *Dr. Jonathan Davidorf*

Can I Wear Contact Lenses after Surgery, If Necessary?

After surgery, if you still need correction in one or both eyes, you may elect to wear contact lenses. With LASIK, you may wear contacts within a few weeks. If you had no previous problems with contacts before LASIK, it is doubtful you will have problems afterward. Realistically, however, rather than returning you to contact lens wear, your surgeon will likely recommend an enhancement to sharpen your vision.

Could the Surgery Cause Problems Years from Now?

The chance of problems years down the road is very unlikely. LASIK is a form of lamellar refractive surgery, a type of surgery that has been performed since 1949. It's important to know that patients who have undergone earlier types of lamellar refractive surgery—much less accurate and more invasive than LASIK—have not developed any unusual problems during the past fifty years.

Will Having LASIK Prevent Eye Diseases?

No. LASIK does not prevent cataracts, glaucoma, retinal detachment, macular degeneration, or any other eye disease. Eye doctors refer to LASIK as *disease neutral*. That is, LASIK does not prevent diseases, and if you are diagnosed with a disease in the future, LASIK will not affect its treatment.

Are There New Developments I Should Know About?

Most doctors keep up with the latest technology and research in their field. Some attend conferences and lectures. Others immerse themselves in a lifestyle that includes lecturing, writing journal articles and textbooks, participating in clinical trials for new technology, and consulting for ophthalmology companies. Find out if there's any news that might impact your decision to have LASIK surgery.

Should I Have Both Eyes Done at the Same Time?

Some patients choose to have one eye treated at a time, because they worry, "What if something goes wrong?" These patients can have the other eye done as soon as a week later. However, our practice as surgeons is generally to do both eyes on the same day. We are extremely confident about the safety of LASIK, and none of us have had a patient lose vision in either or both eyes from the procedure. Having both eyes done together avoids making two trips to the surgery center and speeds the recovery. Correcting the eyes on separate days leaves you with an interim period of imbalanced vision during which only one eye is corrected. In the end, the choice is yours, and you should feel no pressure to do it one way or the other.

What is Monovision?

For monovision, the surgeon corrects one eye for seeing at a distance and the other eye for near vision, thereby reducing the need for reading glasses. When both eyes are functioning together, the brain naturally selects the image from the eye that has the clearer focus. Monovision is similar to stereo sound, where each ear hears a slightly different pattern of sound, but the brain synthesizes it into a sound field. Having eyes for different purposes might sound unsettling, but many patients do quite well with monovision.

You may wish to discuss monovision with your surgeon if you are in your forties or older. As mentioned earlier, patients approaching middle age begin to develop presbyopia, or difficulty with their fine (close-up) focusing. Patients over the age of forty who have both eyes corrected for distance with LASIK will still eventually need reading glasses to see nearby objects.

Disadvantages of monovision include some loss of depth perception and the possibility of impaired night vision. Monovision may not be a good option for people in certain professions—airplane pilot, bus driver, or professional athlete, for example. Some people also find monovision difficult to get used to. Discuss it with your doctor. He or she may be able to show you with contact lenses what monovision would feel like before you have to make a firm decision.

If you do try monovision and do not like it, you can have an enhancement procedure to make the vision in both eyes equal. Ideally, though, it would be better to make this decision beforehand, to avoid an additional procedure.

Informed Consent

If your doctor determines, based on the examination, that you are a candidate for LASIK, he or she will ask you to sign an informed consent form. This is your written legal consent to have the surgeon proceed with your LASIK surgery. Review it carefully, and sign it only after you understand everything on the form. Don't be shy about asking questions.

Working with Your Eye Doctor

Many primary eye doctors today offer LASIK surgery as an option for their patients who don't want to wear glasses or contact lenses. If you have a good primary eye doctor, he or she will review the risks and complications of LASIK with you and provide written material to further your education. He or she will often do the comprehensive eye examination to ensure your eyes are healthy, and then refer you to a capable surgeon. Often the primary doctor will also provide routine postoperative care for you as well. This carefully coordinated sharing of care between the surgeon and your primary eye doctor is called comanagement. It offers you the advantage of a second expert who knows you well to oversee the process and ensure that you are satisfied with the results.

5

Wavefront Technology:
How It Has Improved LASIK

During your consultation, you may be offered a newer diagnostic procedure, known as wavefront analysis. Wavefront technology was first developed for high-powered telescopes, to sharpen the image of distant stars that were distorted by the earth's atmosphere.

More recently, the technology has been applied to the correction of human vision. In 2002, the U.S. Food and Drug Administration approved the use of wavefront-guided LASIK surgery, also known as Custom LASIK. This technology allows the surgeon to custom sculpt the cornea, correcting vision problems more accurately and with fewer side effects.

Wavefront: A Better Diagnostic Tool

The advantage to wavefront-guided LASIK is that it does a much better job of diagnosing the aberrations in your eyes. Traditional LASIK measurements are based on only one point in the eye and correct lower-order aberrations. However, wavefront analysis measures 200 different points in the eye, providing a much better map of the eye's imperfections, including higher-order aberrations. As noted in chapter 1, higher-order aberrations include problems with visual crispness, clarity, and sensitivity contrast. With the data from the wavefront analysis, the

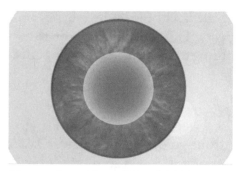

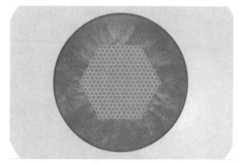

Diagnostics with traditional LASIK measure aberrations at one point in the eye, as shown above.

Wavefront analysis measures 200 points in the eye, providing a better map of the eye's imperfections.

ophthalmologist can now perform LASIK surgery that detects, measures, and corrects both low-order and higher-order aberrations.

How Does Wavefront Analysis Work?

When your surgeon assesses your eye's imperfections with wavefront technology, he or she will probably use the most common wavefront technique—the Hartmann-Shack wavefront sensing method. During this process, your surgeon will shine a low-powered laser into your eye and will ask you to focus on the light. As the light is reflected out of your eye, an aberrometer, a sensing device with many small lenses, will precisely measure your eye's unique cluster of imperfections.

These data are translated into a constellation of "spots," and a special camera will take a picture of them. The data are then compared with the way light travels through eyes that have perfect vision. The difference between these two measurements is used to create a three-dimensional wavefront map.

Once this map, or blueprint, of the eye is produced, it is converted into a mathematical formula and fed into a computer. Later, this information is used to guide the laser beam as it reshapes your cornea during LASIK or PRK surgery. This allows the surgeon to customize your laser treatment according to the precise visual imperfections unique to your eye.

Better Results with Wavefront

Patients who undergo wavefront-guided LASIK have a faster recovery, sharper vision, and fewer side effects. A study at the Naval Medical Center in San Diego compared the results of Navy patients who had had conventional LASIK with the results of those who had had wavefront-guided LASIK.

The results of the study indicated that 88 percent of conventional LASIK patients had achieved 20/20 or better vision six months after surgery. In contrast, 97 percent of the wavefront-guided LASIK patients had achieved 20/20 or better vision after the same time period.

Thirty percent of conventional LASIK patients reported an increase in seeing halos around lights at night, especially when driving. (This can be a temporary side effect of LASIK surgery). None

---

**Benefits of Wavefront-Guided LASIK
Compared to Conventional LASIK**

- Greater chance of achieving 20/20 vision
- Higher quality of vision
- Possible correction of irregular corneas from previous surgeries
- Decreased need for enhancement procedures
- Decreased risk of complications such as night glare and halos

of the wavefront-guided LASIK patients reported this side effect.

Overall, the study concluded that wavefront-guided LASIK offers patients better quality of vision than conventional LASIK, because it significantly decreases night vision problems, such as halos or glare. Wavefront patients reported a greater level of satisfaction with their results than the conventional group did.

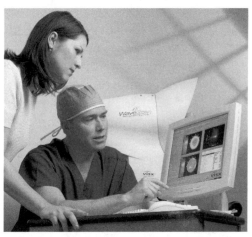

Who Is a Candidate for Wavefront?

Most people who are candidates for conventional LASIK are also candidates for wavefront-guided LASIK. Should everyone

Dr. Robert Maloney discusses a patient's wavefront analysis, which measures visual imperfections in the eyes. The analysis is then used to guide the laser during the LASIK procedure. (*Photo courtesy of Advanced Medical Optical.*)

have a wavefront analysis, especially in light of the fact that it may involve an additional cost and some individuals may get an excellent result with conventional LASIK? Many eye doctors recommend it to all patients who are candidates, because the evidence is that, on average, it produces better vision than conventional treatment for all patients.

Individuals who have problems with image contrast or night vision while wearing their glasses or contacts may be especially interested in wavefront technology, because it can be effective in treating these visual errors.

Some patients who have already undergone an eye treatment may also be candidates; see the section on "Therapeutic Wavefront-Guided Retreatment."

Who Is Not a Candidate for Wavefront?

Even though wavefront is an advancement in LASIK, it is not for everyone. Because wavefront involves the removal of more corneal tissue than conventional LASIK, individuals with thin corneas may not be candidates. If you have small pupils you may not be a candidate because the wavefront measurements require a minimum pupil size for accuracy. For technical reasons, in some people the traditional measurements are more accurate than the wavefront measurements. Your surgeon will recommend the method of measurement that gives you the best chance of excellent vision.

Potential Complications

The risks of wavefront-guided LASIK are the same as the risks of conventional LASIK. Further details of potential risks are covered in chapter 8.

However, it is important to note that wavefront-guided LASIK may actually prevent some of the side effects that occur more often with conventional LASIK. Some patients who undergo conventional LASIK have problems with glare or halos around lights at night or in dim lighting. These side effects usually occur because conventional LASIK can increase some higher-order aberrations. Because wavefront-guided LASIK is designed to correct these higher-order aberrations, such side effects are less likely to occur.

Cost for Wavefront

Wavefront-guided laser surgery is more expensive than conventional LASIK. The price varies among geographical locations and among surgeons. As with conventional LASIK, the fact that insurance companies consider this type of surgery "cosmetic" means they often will not cover the cost. Many surgeons offer financing options, however.

Therapeutic Wavefront-Guided Retreatment

Wavefront technology is helpful in retreating problems that may result from LASIK. Occasionally, patients develop problems with quality of nighttime or daytime vision after undergoing LASIK surgery. These problems are usually caused by higher-order aberrations. Therapeutic wavefront-guided retreatment is a process employed by experienced surgeons during which wavefront technology is used to measure these higher-order aberrations; then the data gleaned from the wavefront technology are used to perform a LASIK retreatment. This application of wavefront technology can be used to treat many potential LASIK side effects, such as halos, multiple images, undercorrection, and glare.

6

Undergoing LASIK

On the day of your LASIK procedure, it is natural to experience both excitement and nervousness. Patients who feel most at ease on that day are those who have asked questions, read about the LASIK procedure, and perhaps talked with former patients. Understanding LASIK and trusting your surgeon are important to helping you feel confident, calm, and prepared on the day of your procedure.

You won't be able to drive immediately after the procedure, so it is recommended that you have someone drive you to the surgery center and pick you up when you're ready to leave.

Arriving at the Center

Make an effort to arrive at the center rested and relaxed. You should plan to spend one and a half to three hours at the laser center, although this amount of time varies from center to center.

Wear comfortable clothing the day of your surgery. Do not wear makeup, skin moisturizer, perfume, or cologne because LASIK requires clean, sterile conditions. Earrings should not be worn either.

How the LASIK Procedure Is Performed

LASIK is performed while the patient is awake. However, if you are experiencing anxiety, the surgeon may give you a mild oral sedative. Many surgeons talk to the patient throughout the procedure so the individual knows what is happening and what to expect next.

Before the Procedure

Before the surgery begins, your face will be cleaned with a disinfectant, and you will be asked to wear a surgical cap. You will be given eyedrops, which may sting for a few seconds.

Undergoing the Procedure

Once in the laser suite, you will be positioned comfortably on your back, under the excimer laser. Your surgeon will give you anesthetic eyedrops to numb the surface of your eyes. Your eyelashes will be taped out of the way,

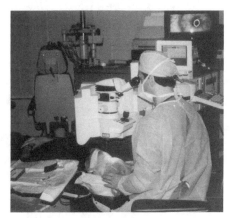

LASIK surgery, performed here by Dr. Ernest Kornmehl, is an out-patient procedure.

and an *eyelid speculum* will be placed between your eyelids to keep you from blinking. The speculum sometimes causes mild pressure on your eyelids at first, but with the numbing drops, these sensations dissipate.

A suction ring is then placed on your eye to hold it in position while the flap is made. Your vision will dim during this step. The surgeon will then use the microkeratome to create the corneal flap. The microkeratome is a precision instrument that automatically peels back the outer layers of cornea, creating a flap that is thinner than a soft contact lens. The extremely thin flap is made from the outermost 25 percent of the cornea. The average cornea, remember, is only about the thickness of a credit card. This flap-making process takes about fifteen seconds. When the microkeratome is making the flap, you may feel slight pressure, and the instrument will block out light as it passes over your pupil.

Next, the surgeon will ask you to fix your vision on a target light —usually red, green, or yellow. Then the surgeon will gently lift back the hinged flap. At this point your vision will become blurry.

The surgeon will now perform the laser procedure. This usually takes twenty to ninety seconds. You will not feel any pain as the laser sculpts the cornea by vaporizing small amounts of tissue. This process is called *photoablation*. You will also hear a clicking or buzzing sound with each pulse of the laser. The surgeon is reshaping your cornea.

If you're in the hands of a competent surgeon, the incidence of serious complications is remote, so it's important that patients are sure they've found a good surgeon.

Dr. Jonathan Davidorf

The best lasers today have eye tracking devices that follow your eye during the laser treatment. As mentioned earlier, this provides an extra level of safety. If you move your eye during the treatment, the laser follows your eye.

Once the process of reshaping your corneal tissue is complete, the excimer laser will be turned off. Using a sterile saline solution, the surgeon will flush the treated surface of the eye to ensure that any debris is washed away. The surgeon will then carefully replace the corneal flap to its original position.

It takes about one to five minutes for the eye to create a natural vacuum to hold down the flap. The cornea has the unique ability to seal itself back in place. The flap adheres like Velcro, so no sutures are necessary. The eyelid speculum will be removed. You will now be able to blink normally.

At this point, you will be asked to sit with your eyes closed for about thirty minutes. Then your eyes will be examined one more time to ensure that the corneal flap is properly positioned.

LASIK Step-by-Step

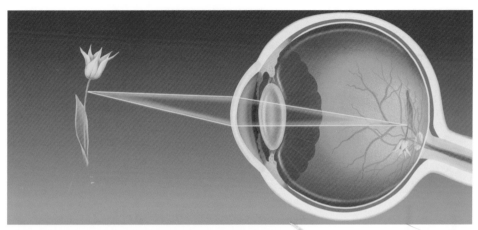

Normal refraction is shown here. Light passes through the cornea and focuses properly on the retina. The result is a clear image of the flower.

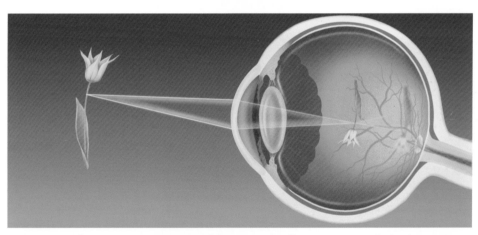

A patient with myopia is represented here. As the flower is viewed, the image is focused in front of the retina, near the middle of the eyeball. As a result, the image that forms on the retina is blurred, as shown by the flower on the right.

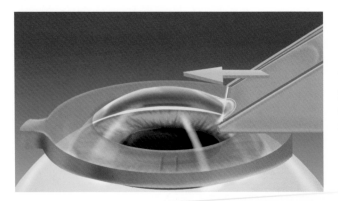

The fine blade of the microkeratome begins to create the thin corneal flap.

The microkeratome continues to advance across the cornea, creating the corneal flap.

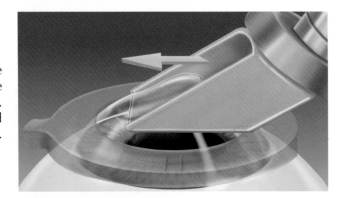

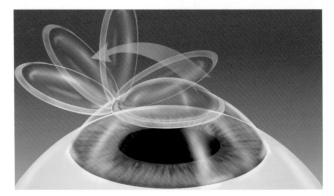

The corneal flap is folded back to expose the bed of the corneal stroma.

The prepared corneal bed is now ready for treatment with the excimer laser.

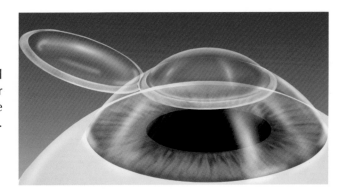

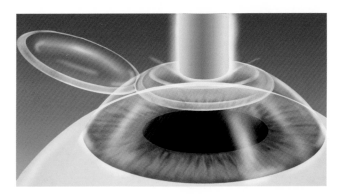

The cool laser beam ablates and reshapes the cornea.

Configuration of the cornea after laser treatment. The laser was preprogrammed to reduce (flatten) the curvature of the cornea.

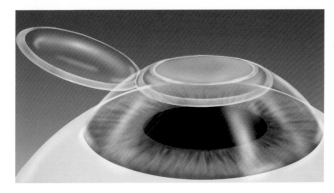

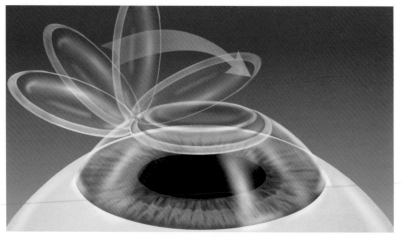

The corneal flap is replaced over the treated corneal stroma. No sutures are required.

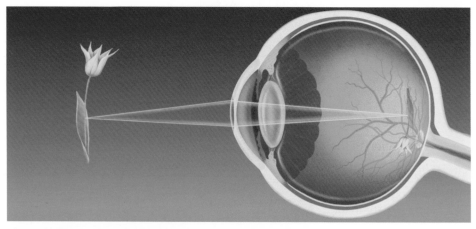

The refraction is corrected for the myopic patient. The subtle change of the reshaped cornea is shown in purple at the front of the eyeball.

Patients who have undergone LASIK may experience some discomfort, which may last six to eight hours. Patients describe this as a sensation of having sand or a dirty contact lens in their eye. Acetaminophen, aspirin, ibuprofen, or similar over-the-counter pain medications can help. By bedtime the night of surgery, this sensation is usually gone.

Immediately after surgery, expect your vision to be somewhat blurred, similar to looking through a glass of water or wearing a dirty contact lens. However, upon awakening later in the day or the next morning, you will experience improved vision. Most patients report dramatic improvement within twenty-four hours.

Going Home

When you are ready to go home, you will receive antibiotic drops, anti-inflammatory drops to promote healing, and lubricating eyedrops, also called "artificial tears." It is common for the eyes to feel somewhat dry after LASIK. You will be sent home with detailed instructions on the use of the various eyedrops. You will wear clear plastic shields or goggles over your eyes for several hours after surgery and while you sleep that night. These eye shields prevent accidental trauma to the corneal flap during the healing period, in case you inadvertently bump your eye while you are sleeping.

Your surgeon will probably advise that you go home and take a nap. You may be given a mild sedative to make you sleepy. It is best to have your eyes closed for the first few hours after surgery, and sleep is the easiest way to accomplish this.

7

After Your LASIK Procedure

Within hours of your surgery, constantly regenerating cells will already be growing over the edge of the corneal flap, helping to "glue" it down. This process takes a few days. Over the next several months, the internal healing process will totally seal the flap.

In the interim, however, it's important that you do all you can to make the surgery a success. The moment you leave the LASIK center, you are encouraged to take an active role in your body's healing process by following a specific regimen prescribed by your eye doctor.

Who Performs Your Postoperative Care?

You may have a choice of having your postoperative care performed by the surgeon (or another doctor on his staff) or your regular eye doctor. If you are traveling far to be treated by an expert surgeon, you will naturally want to have your eye doctor close to home take care of you. If the surgeon is located nearby, you may still wish to have your regular eye doctor provide your routine postoperative care.

Your eye doctor will check your vision and examine your eyes to ensure proper healing, and he or she can provide temporary eyeglasses or contact lenses if needed during the healing process. After you have healed, he or she can also help you make the decision about whether or not enhancement is appropriate if your vision is not perfect. Your regular eye doctor will stay in close contact with the surgeon in case any difficulties arise during your postoperative course.

Your Self-Care Regimen

Follow these recommended guidelines to promote safe and rapid healing.

- Rest or sleep for the first four hours after surgery with your eyes closed. This helps the flap remain smooth while it develops a tight adherence to the underlying tissue.

- Keep your eyes well lubricated for rapid recovery and enhanced comfort. Particularly in dry climates or air-conditioned environments, you may need to apply nonpreserved lubricant eye-drops frequently. Some patients may need these drops every couple of hours for a few weeks after surgery. Your surgeon will recommend a good brand.

- Wear high-quality sunglasses with ultraviolet protection. It is normal to experience increased sensitivity to light at first. This condition will improve.

- Avoid rubbing your eyes for a few days. The corneal flap needs time to adhere evenly without being disturbed.

- Avoid rough contact sports for the first week, for the same reason.

- Avoid swimming, surfing, and hot tubs for one week to prevent contact with unwanted germs and bacteria that could cause infection before the corneal flap has totally healed.

- Showers and baths are fine, but for the first few days, be careful to avoid getting water and shampoo directly in your eyes.

- Avoid dusty or smoky environments for several days.
- Avoid wearing old mascara and eyeliner for one week.
- Don't drive on the day of surgery. Resume driving only when your vision is clear enough that you are safe on the road. Most people easily see well enough to drive safely the morning after surgery, but it may be a few days before you feel comfortable enough to drive.

I think LASIK is the tip of the iceberg. I believe eyeglasses will be totally obsolete in twenty years. Our grandvhildren will look at eyeglasses the way we look at monocles and whalebone girdles.

Dr. Robert Maloney

Postoperative Appointment Schedule

Keeping your follow-up appointments is important, even if your vision is perfect. Your doctor needs to follow the progress of your healing and may recommend changing your eyedrop regimen. Also, he or she may need to monitor your eye pressure if you are on postoperative anti-inflammatory drops for any length of time; these drops may increase pressure inside the eye, creating a risk for glaucoma.

The LASIK Recovery Cycle

Most patients are genuinely surprised by how quickly their vision improves after LASIK. Although the corneal flap adheres quickly, your eyesight will continue to improve until it finally reaches a point at which it becomes stable. The time it takes to establish visual stability after LASIK varies for each patient. For some, stability can be achieved in a few weeks. For others, stability may take three to six months.

During the first month after surgery, you will probably notice a gradual improvement in your vision. It is common to experience fluctuations in your vision during the first two to three weeks, especially for those with higher corrections.

Patients who have hyperopic LASIK (farsightedness treatment) may notice that at first their near vision is better than their distance vision. This is quite common, and the distance vision will continue to improve during the first month.

For the first three months, it is normal for patients to experience an occasional feeling of "grittiness" in the eye. This is related to dryness on the surface of the eye. Using lubricating eyedrops will help significantly. People with drier eyes and those who use a computer, read for long hours, drive long distances, or live in low-humidity climates may even notice some minor discomfort and blurring of their vision, particularly toward the end of the day. Also caused by dryness, these conditions will improve over time.

Although many patients notice halos around lights or ghosting of images at night, these symptoms tend to lessen substantially within six months.

Before your vision stabilizes, you may feel more comfortable with a thin pair of eyeglasses—those with low prescription lenses—to assist you with critical distance vision activities, such as driving at night. Patients over forty years of age may require a thin pair of glasses for reading.

8

Risks and Complications

Just as all surgical procedures carry risks, so does the LASIK procedure. However, when LASIK is performed by an experienced surgeon, the risk of complications is quite low. In fact, this surgery is among the safest performed today.

Still, it's important to understand the risks and possible complications. Once you understand them, you will be able to determine for yourself whether the potential benefits of laser vision correction outweigh the risks.

Improper Screening

Most complications are preventable. One of the most common reasons for complications following surgery is improper screening of the surgery candidate. An inexperienced surgeon may fail to detect a condition that would make you a poor candidate, whereas an experienced surgeon may advise you against having LASIK, after having performed a careful preoperative examination. As discussed earlier, there are many reasons to turn down a patient. That is why it's important to choose a surgeon based on his or her competence—not on the cheapest fee available.

Possible Complications
Undercorrection

Undercorrection results when the desired change in your refractive error, or focusing ability, is not fully achieved after the LASIK procedure. A slight undercorrection will not seriously affect your vision and may even be desirable in nearsighted patients over forty to help with their reading vision. More significant undercorrections may require an enhancement procedure, which sometimes included in the original LASIK cost if performed within the first year.

Undercorrection happens more often in patients with higher levels of nearsightedness, farsightedness, or astigmatism. This makes sense if you think in terms of how much sculpting, or reshaping, the laser has to do. For example, a patient with less than 2.00 diopters of myopia has about a 1 percent chance of needing an enhancement procedure because of an undercorrection. On the other hand, a patient with more than 9.00 diopters of myopia has about a 10 percent chance of requiring an enhancement procedure due to undercorrection.

Surgeons who use consistent techniques and constantly analyze their outcomes have significantly lower incidences of undercorrection. This is another reason it is important to find a surgeon who tracks LASIK outcomes, as discussed earlier. If your doctor keeps an up-to-date database of at least 1,000 procedures, he or she will be able to show you the likelihood of your needing retreatment, based on your own degree and type of refractive error.

Overcorrection

Overcorrection results when the refractive error is changed more than was intended. An initial, or temporary, overcorrection may occur and usually rights itself in the first month. After a treatment for far-sightedness, an overcorrection would make you temporarily near-sighted. In this case, your distance vision would be somewhat blurred and your near vision rather good. Following a treatment for nearsight-edness, an overcorrection would make it more difficult for you to see objects up close. Patients can manage a temporary overcorrection by wearing glasses until it resolves.

There are fewer permanent overcorrections than permanent under-corrections. A significant overcorrection can be treated with an enhance-ment procedure as well. An overcorrection enhancement is usually performed three to six months after the initial treatment, once the patient's vision has stabilized.

Induced Astigmatism

In rare circumstances, significant astigmatism results after the ini-tial LASIK surgery. *Induced astigmatism* causes blurred vision. It can be treated with enhancement surgery, if it is bothersome. Most peo-ple can tolerate small degrees of astigmatism. However, if your vision is blurred because of a refractive error after LASIK and does not meet your expectations, there is a 99 percent chance that it can be correct-ed with enhancement.

Dry Eye

As detailed earlier, it is not uncommon for patients to experi-ence a feeling of dryness or grittiness in the eye after LASIK. This is a common side effect from the surgery that will usually decrease over the first few weeks. The use of nonpreserved lubricating eye-drops (artificial tears), punctual plugs, or a medication called *Restasis* will help alleviate the symptoms of dry eye.

LASIK makes the eyes somewhat drier than before surgery. For most patients this is not a problem, because the eyes have more moisture than needed; so a little dryness is not bothersome. However, in rare cases patients develop more significant dryness after LASIK. These patients experience dryness throughout the day. You are more at risk for this if you have dry eyes before LASIK when wearing glasses. (Many people have dry eyes while wearing contact lenses, but this is not a risk factor if the dry eye is treated before the LASIK procedure.) An important part of the comprehensive examination is an evaluation of tears to ensure that your chance of experiencing post-LASIK dryness is minimal. If you do develop persistent dryness, a variety of treatments are now available. These include taking dietary supplements, using lubricating eyedrops, using eyedrops that improve tear production, and blocking your tear drainage canals with tiny plugs to retain more tears in your eyes.

> *Patients need to understand LASIK's potential risks as well as the benefits. Prior to performing the procedure, I need to know that the patient truly wants the surgery, rather than having a spouse or significant other pushing them into it.*
>
> *Dr. Ernest Kornmehl*

Corneal Abrasion

Approximately 1 to 5 percent of LASIK patients develop a small *corneal abrasion*, or scrape, caused by friction of the microkeratome. The eye is covered by a thin layer of skin, called the epithelium. This skin is just like the skin on your hand except that it is clear so you can see through it. Occasionally, the minor trauma of surgery causes part of the epithelium to fall away. This is called a corneal abrasion or corneal epithelial defect. This doesn't harm your eye and doesn't interfere with the laser treatment. However, your eye will be uncomfortable while the epithelium heals, just as your hand is after it is scraped.

Your surgeon will know immediately if you develop a corneal abrasion when the LASIK procedure is performed on your eye; he or she will place a very thin contact lens on the eye. This is called a bandage lens, because it serves as a protective layer over the eye surface.

The lens increases comfort and promotes healing. It can be removed in one to five days. The abrasions always heal, usually in one to three days. But it may take up to ten days to achieve your best vision if the abrasion is located centrally.

While the abrasion is healing, your vision will be blurred—as if you were looking through a scratched pair of eyeglasses. In rare cases, if the corneal abrasion is significant, the surgeon may decide to postpone doing LASIK on the other eye for one or two weeks, giving the first eye a chance to heal. Postponement of surgery on the second eye ensures that you don't have blurry vision in both eyes at the same time.

Night Glare and Halos

All people, whether or not they have had LASIK, experience some glare or halos at night. These night-vision disturbances occur when you are in a dark environment and look at a small bright light, such as a headlight or a streetlight. *Halo* is the glow that surrounds the light source, and *glare* is little spikes of light that appear to emanate from the light source like the rays around a light. Glare and halos occur because the pupil dilates in low-light conditions. The dilated pupil allows more peripheral light rays (rays coming in from the sides) to enter the eye. These rays are more likely to scatter, instead of coming to a precise focus. You perceive the scattered light as glare or halos. Incidentally, this scattering of light from proper focus is why everyone notices that his or her night vision is not as good as their daytime vision.

Some patients experience an increase in these symptoms after LASIK. Although these symptoms do not necessarily interfere with visual sharpness as measured on the Snellen eye chart, they can be bothersome in dim-light conditions, such as driving at night. Some patients may see glare and halos at night during the first month after treatment; however, it is quite uncommon for these side effects to interfere with patients' activities. The effects usually improve in the first three months, and the overwhelming majority of significant glare problems disappear on their own by six months. There are treatment options for patients who experience persistent glare or halos. Weak prescription night glasses can help, as can the use at dusk of eyedrops that reduce the size of the pupils. Wavefront-guided retreatment is also a promising approach.

It's difficult to predict one patient's chances of having these symptoms after LASIK. Patients with more severe refractive errors and astigmatism may be more prone to glare and halo effects. Many eye doctors used to believe that patients with larger pupils had a greater chance of developing glare or halos at night, although a number of major studies have now shown that this is not true. Special programs for the laser that allow for larger treatment zones can help reduce the chance of these problems.

The newer wavefront-guided laser treatment has been shown to significantly reduce night-vision disturbances compared with conventional laser treatment, which is another reason many surgeons recommend it to all eligible patients.

Problems with Quality of Vision

A small number of patients experience a slight loss of quality of vision after LASIK surgery. This is also called *loss of best-corrected vision*. Loss of best-corrected vision means that, even with eyeglasses, a patient loses some of the visual crispness and clarity he or she had when wearing eyeglasses or contacts prior to surgery. The person may no longer be able to read the 20/20 line on the Snellen eye chart. He or she may also notice some hazy vision or ghost images. Loss of best-corrected vision can be a result of irregular healing or an irregular flap and may improve over the first year. This complication is very rare except in those with very high levels of nearsightness or astigmatism. Careful surgical technique and good follow-up care help minimize the incidence of this problem.

Development of a "Central Island"

Another potential complication from LASIK is the development of a *central island*, a small raised area in the cornea's treatment zone. Central islands often disappear spontaneously after several months, but some require an enhancement procedure; in this, the corneal flap is lifted and a small amount of excimer laser energy is delivered to the raised area. When the central island is removed by additional laser treatment, crisp vision usually returns.

The surgeon diagnoses a central island by using a corneal topographer, the device that produces a digitized contour map of the corneal surface. To help prevent central islands, some excimer lasers have special software that distributes additional pulses centrally, along with the regular treatment for the refractive error. With the latest generation of excimer lasers, the incidence of central islands is very low.

Corneal Flap Complications

For experienced surgeons, corneal flap complications are rare, occurring in about 1 in 2,000 procedures. This complication is characterized by a flap that is too small, too thin, detached, or irregularly shaped. After the surgeon makes the flap, he or she inspects it. If there are problems with the flap, the surgeon may not proceed with the laser treatment. He or she will replace the flap and terminate the operation. Typically, vision quickly returns to the way it was before surgery. While this complication is frightening, it almost never harms vision if the surgeon handles the problem correctly. The LASIK procedure can usually be successfully repeated in six months, after the eye heals.

Striae

Sometimes the corneal flap may shift slightly in the first twelve hours after LASIK surgery. This is why it is important, especially during the first few hours, not to rub your eyes and to keep them well lubricated. If the flap shifts slightly, wrinkles form, just as wrinkles form in a carpet if you step on it and it isn't properly nailed down. The medical term for these wrinkles is *striae*. If striae are present in the center of the cornea, they may blur your vision. Fortunately, striae are easy to fix with a brief, painless procedure if treated early. The flap is lifted and laid back down smoothly, and the surgeon places a clear bandage contact lens, that holds the flap securely in place, to wear overnight.

Epithelial Ingrowth

The cornea is covered by a thin, clear skin, called epithelium. This clear skin is made of epithelial cells. When the LASIK flap is lifted and replaced, these cells normally grow back over the top of the flap. About 1 percent of the time, the cells grow under the flap instead. This condition is called *epithelial ingrowth*. These cells occasionally cause blurred vision or irritation. Epithelial ingrowth is easy to identify and is treated by gently lifting the flap and clearing away the trapped epithelial cells. Epithelial ingrowth is more common following enhancement procedures when the original flap is relifted.

Regression

Regression refers to the tendency of the eye to drift back slightly toward the original refractive error. This occurs more commonly in patients with higher degrees of myopia, hyperopia, or astigmatism.

If significant regression occurs, you may require either low-prescription eyeglasses for night driving or an enhancement procedure to "tune up" the original treatment, provided your cornea is thick enough to allow retreatment. Enhancements for regression are usually performed three to six months after the original procedure, to allow time for the patient's vision to stabilize.

Diffuse Lamellar Keratitis

This condition, *diffuse lamellar keratitis* (DLK)—also known as "sands of the Sahara" syndrome—is an inflammation that occurs in the space between the corneal flap and the underlying stroma. This relatively rare condition is typically observed by the doctor the day after surgery. You may have no symptoms, or you may notice some haziness in your vision or a mild irritation. After LASIK, all patients are given a topical corticosteroid, a medicated eyedrop used to suppress inflammation. You will be instructed to apply these drops at least four days after the procedure. These drops prevent DLK from occurring in the great majority of patients.

There is considerable debate about what causes DLK. It is normally easily treated with topical corticosteroids. Most cases of DLK respond promptly to this treatment. More severe cases may require that the surgeon lift the corneal flap and irrigate beneath it to remove the inflammatory cells. Severe cases may cause some blurring of vision that necessitates an enhancement procedure, although these cases are extraordinarily rare. When recognized early and treated properly, DLK resolves quickly.

Keratoconus and Corneal Ectasia

Keratoconus is a naturally occurring disease caused by a weakness in the cornea. Keratoconus naturally occurs in some people as they age. Patients with this condition suffer from increasingly poor vision as their corneas bulge and thin over time due to the pressure put on their weakened corneas. Symptoms often reported by keratoconus patients include nearsightedness and fluctuating vision (irregular astigmatism). This disease is progressive, but does not progress much after age forty. Scientists are not completely sure of the causes of keratoconus, but genetics is believed to play a large part.

Patients who suffer from preexisting keratoconus are not candidates for LASIK, because LASIK in some cases accelerates the progression of the disease. An essential part of your consultation is examining you for keratoconus, using a specialized diagnostic map of the eye called *corneal topography*.

Corneal ectasia is a disorder that appears just like keratoconus but develops after LASIK. It is also called *secondary keratoconus* or *iatrogenic keratoconus*. It is very rare, and its causes are uncertain. Some patients who develop ectasia after LASIK would have developed keratoconus even without LASIK surgery because of their genetic predisposition. Other patients develop it because the surgeon removed too much tissue during the procedure. Poor preoperative screening is often a factor in these cases. To prevent ectasia after LASIK, your surgeon will measure your corneal thickness before surgery. He or she should ensure that you have a minimum of 220 to 250 microns of tissue remaining after LASIK.

Corneal ectasia is very rare. Those who are at higher risk for developing ectasia include people with extreme myopia or whose eyes have an irregular preoperative shape or people who have a particularly thin cornea. It is important to note that corneal ectasia has occurred in patients with no risk factors and after LASIK procedures that appeared to be free of complications.

In its early stages, keratoconus and ectasia are often successfully managed with rigid gas permeable contact lenses. Patients often find they are able to use these lenses for many years with few problems. *Intacs*, tiny rings inserted into the cornea to correct nearsightedness, are also used to manage keratoconus in early stages of treatment. In more advanced cases, keratoconus may require a corneal transplant. Patients who cannot wear the rigid gas permeable contact lens may also need a transplant. Usually, corneal transplants are very successful. Unlike keratoconus, corneal ectasia is not usually progressive, so even patients who develop it do not usually require a corneal transplant.

Infection

Although infection is the most feared complication, it is extremely rare, occurring in about 1 in 10,000 surgeries done by an experienced surgeon. As with any surgery, proper technique is the best way to avoid infection. If your eye does become infected, it will likely occur during the first forty-eight to seventy-two hours after LASIK. This is why it is so important for the first week to avoid any contact with substances that may cause infection, such as eye makeup, hot tubs, and swimming pools. It is also essential to go to all of your follow-up visits, even if everything seems fine. To prevent infection, you will use antibiotic drops postoperatively for a few days to a week.

9

PRK

Although you may not be a candidate for LASIK, the most popular refractive procedure performed today, you may be a candidate for a procedure known as photorefractive keractectomy, or PRK. This procedure delivers the same visual outcomes as LASIK and has dramatically improved the vision of millions of patients unable to undergo the LASIK procedure.

What is PRK?

Like LASIK, PRK is refractive surgical procedure which uses a laser to reshape the cornea. However, rather than creating a flap and then reshaping the deeper corneal layers, PRK uses the same excimer laser to sculpt directly on the surface layers of the cornea. You can think of PRK as LASIK without the flap. For mild to moderate myopia, only 5 to 10 percent of the thickness of the cornea is removed; for extreme myopia, about 30 percent of cornea thickness is removed. If you were to measure this tissue, its thickness would be that of one to three human hairs. The major benefit of PRK is that the structure of the corneal dome is retained.

The PRK procedure also goes by several other names: LASEK (pronounced LAS-ECK), epi-LASIK, and surface ablation.

History of PRK

As mentioned earlier in this book, PRK was introduced in 1987 and was approved by the U.S. FDA in 1995. Instead of a microkeratome being used to create a corneal flap, with PRK the surgeon uses the laser to accurately sculpt the cornea one microscopic layer at a time. As awareness of LASIK grew, PRK became less popular, because of the increased comfort and more rapid recovery of vision that LASIK offered.

In the last decade, a newer generation of excimer lasers, along with refined techniques, have minimized the risks of PRK. And patients today have an easier recovery. As a result, PRK has become a viable option for a variety of patients whose needs are not met by LASIK.

Who Is a Candidate for PRK?

Most people who are candidates for LASIK are also candidates for PRK. The PRK procedure is an especially good fit for people with mild to moderate nearsightedness, farsightedness, and/or astigmatism. Individuals with thin corneas may be better candidates for PRK than for LASIK. As with any laser surgery, your corneas should be healthy and your vision should be stable for at least a year prior to the procedure. Also, except in certain situations, you need to be at least eighteen years of age to undergo this procedure.

Who Is Not a Candidate for PRK?

If you have herpes simplex of the eye, you cannot undergo the procedure during an active outbreak. Some doctors will do PRK if you go six months without a recurrence of herpes. In this case, you will need prophylactic medications before and after the procedure to minimize the risk of a recurrence while the eye heals.

In general, pregnant women should avoid vision correction procedures, including PRK, because pregnancy sometimes causes instability in one's prescription during the third trimester. On the other hand, if you are early in your pregnancy and your vision hasn't changed, it may be possible to do PRK in special cases.

You may be surprised to learn that if you suffer from major medical conditions—an autoimmune disease, such as lupus or rheumatoid arthritis, or diabetes for example—you are not automatically disqualified for PRK surgery. Talk with your surgeon about specific steps you can take to make PRK as safe as possible for you.

Surgeon Qualifications

As with LASIK surgery, you'll want to find an ophthalmologist who is board certified. Surgeons who have completed at least 200 PRK procedures should be competent with the procedure.

Preparing for PRK

As with LASIK, you will be asked not to wear contact lenses for up to a week prior to the date of your measurements in order to give your eyes time to return to their natural shape and provide a more accurate correction. If you wear rigid gas permeable contact lenses, your surgeon may request that you not wear them for up to three weeks prior to your measurements for the same reason.

Whether to operate the same day on both eyes or to have each eye treated on different dates is a decision to be made by the patient after discussing the pros and cons with the surgeon. Because the return of functional vision is prolonged after PRK, some prefer to wait at least one week before operating on the second eye. The major drawback is the inconvenience of going through the recovery process (twenty-four to forty-eight hours of pain or discomfort and the postoperative office visits) twice.

You will need to make sure that you have a ride home from your surgeon's office, because you will have been given a mild sedative prior to your procedure.

Your PRK Procedure

On the day of your PRK procedure, make sure that you eat lightly in the morning. You'll also want to avoid wearing eye makeup and any cumbersome hair accessories that could interfere with your surgeon's ability to position your head as needed during your procedure. Also, make sure you wear comfortable clothing for your surgery.

Once in the surgical suite, you are asked to recline under the laser and relax. Your doctor numbs your eye with a topical eyedrop anesthesia. Then, in order to prevent you from blinking during the procedure, he or she will prop your eyelids open with a speculum.

Next, the surgeon gently removes the epithelium, which is the layer of clear "skin" or cells that cover the cornea. The epithelium must be removed because it blocks the laser from reshaping the cornea. The epithelium may be removed with a laser, a blade, a brush, or a special instrument called an epi-keratome. This step differs from the initial step of LASIK surgery, during which the flap is pulled back from the surface to expose the deeper layers of the cornea.

Next, based on measurements your surgeon took during your consultation, he or she will sculpt or reshape the cornea, enabling light to focus properly on the retina. PRK, like LASIK, is performed with an excimer laser, which reshapes the surface of the cornea with its cool, pulsing beam of ultraviolet light. The laser works its way down into the stroma, or structural part of the cornea, where the real reshaping takes place. This part of the procedure takes only twenty to ninety seconds per eye. As the laser removes tissue and reshapes the cornea, you will hear a tapping noise, which is caused by the laser energy.

Once the procedure is complete, a special, clear contact lens, called a *bandage* lens, is placed over your eye to help keep you more comfortable while the corneal epithelium regenerates, usually in three to four days. A typical PRK procedure takes about three to five minutes per eye. The entire process may take up to thirty minutes, though, with the majority of that time devoted to preparing your eyes for surgery.

After Your PRK Procedure

When you sit up in the laser suite after the treatment, you will immediately notice an improvement in your vision. You will be able to return home immediately after surgery. You'll leave the surgeon's office wearing the clear bandage contact lens, through which you can see. Depending on your surgeon's preference, you may be asked to wear an eye shield overnight too.

Do Not Rub Your Eyes

For the first three to five days, avoid rubbing your eyes; doing so could dislodge your contact lens bandage. Also, stay away from swimming pools and hot tubs for at least a week after surgery. The chlorine and other chemicals could irritate your eyes, delay healing, and increase your risk of infection.

Discomfort

Often, patients who have undergone PRK experience twenty-four to forty-eight hours of mild to moderate discomfort until the epithelium regenerates and the surface of the eye regains its smooth contour. Typically, patients report that it feels as if they've scratched their eye. Others report feeling as if they have a grain of sand in their eye. These side effects are normal and should fade as the healing process continues. Meanwhile, to lessen these sensations, you will be given anti-inflammatory drops. You may also be given special anesthetic drops to relieve the pain. Oral pain medications can also be prescribed.

You will also be given antibiotic eyedrops to use for several days to minimize the risk of infection. Do not use any eyedrops that your eye doctor has not approved.

Blurred Vision

Vision typically actually worsens during the first few days while the epithelium regenerates. You will note improved vision that fluctuates quite a bit during the first week after surgery but slowly stabilizes after that.

You may notice that your eyes seem especially sensitive to light. Or you could see more glare or even halos around light at night. Expect that you very well may need to wear glasses for reading or driving for a while after your surgery until your best corrected vision is realized.

The exact timing of achieving good functional vision after PRK is variable and hinges on many factors, including the degree of your correction and the speed at which your eye heals. Some patients are comfortable and functional three days after the procedure, while others may take three to four weeks to be comfortable with their new eyesight.

Resuming Activities

Your surgeon will place very few restrictions on your activities after your surgery. Activities such as exercise, television watching, driving, and flying are all acceptable when you feel up to them. Use common sense and listen to your body to decide which activities are right for you and when you should begin them again.

Follow-up Appointments

Your surgeon will request that you come into the office the day after your procedure. Later, once your corneal surface heals, your surgeon will remove the bandage contact lens in the office. This healing usually takes three to five days. Then the visits to your eye doctor will decrease in frequency to once a week, then once every three weeks, and then every two to three months, to ensure that healing is occurring properly.

Results of Your PRK

Although most PRK patients are already doing quite well at their one-month examination, it may take several months before the entire extent of your vision correction is apparent. Often, patients who are severely nearsighted or farsighted must wait longest for their full results. Your final vision outcome may not be known for certain for a few months, or more, after your procedure. The surface of the eye needs to heal fully before the doctor can actually determine the final results.

PRK Statistics

Published studies demonstrate no difference in the final results between PRK and LASIK at one year after the procedure. As with LASIK, your personal statistics depend on your degree of correction. The smaller your correction, the better the chance of perfect vision. However, even patients with severe nearsightedness report positive results with PRK. Chapter 10 will give you an idea of your chances of 20/20 vision with PRK.

When Retreatment Is Needed

In approximately 5 to 10 percent of PRK cases, a retreatment, or *enhancement*, may be necessary to achieve the optimal level of vision correction you and your surgeon hoped for. During a PRK retreatment, surface cells are removed, and you will experience another one to two days of mild to moderate discomfort. Again, though, you will be prescribed the medication to ease any discomfort. A minimum wait of six months after the original PRK is required for the eyes to become sufficiently stable for laser enhancement.

Potential Complications

In general, the complications of PRK and LASIK are the same. Refer to chapter 8 for a discussion of the complications of LASIK. The information in that chapter applies to PRK, too, with the following differences.

Absence of Flap Complications

One advantage of PRK over LASIK is that there is no risk of flap complications because no corneal flap is created.

Corneal Haze

Corneal haze is clouding of the cornea during the healing process. This clouding may cause blurry or hazy vision. Significant corneal haze following PRK is extremely rare with today's equipment and medications. As a general rule, the worse your eyesight was going into the procedure, the more you are at risk for developing corneal haze. Haze eventually disappears by itself, but this can take months or years. If it develops, corneal haze is usually retreated with the laser to physically remove it, although this is necessary in fewer than 1 percent of patients. Corneal haze does not occur with LASIK.

Comparing PRK with LASIK Surgery
Range of Correction

PRK and LASIK cover the same range of correction—low to moderate farsightedness and low to high nearsightedness with or without astigmatism.

PRK and LASIK: A Comparison

	PRK	LASIK
Range of correction	Low to high	Low to high
Depth of penetration	Superficial 20 percent of corneal depth	Up to 50 percent of corneal depth
Recovery of vision	3 to 5 days	Overnight
Return to work	3 days	Next day
Discomfort during surgery	Minimal or none	Minimal or none
Discomfort after surgery	Mild to moderate for 24–48 hrs	Minimal, 2–4 hours
Postoperative medications	1 week to 3 months	1 week
Time to final vision	1 to 3 months	2 to 4 weeks
Vision achieved	Excellent	Excellent

Depth of Penetration

Because no corneal flap is created, the depth of penetration of PRK into the cornea is less than LASIK. PRK alters only the surface of the cornea. LASIK, on the other hand, penetrates into deeper layers of the cornea.

Recovery of Vision

The recovery from PRK is slower than LASIK. After LASIK, your vision is usually 20/20 or close to it by the next morning. With PRK, vision does not reach this level for 3 to 5 days. Because most of us need to see well in order to perform our jobs, this timeline can be used for going back to work. So, if you have PRK completed in both eyes at the same time, you'll most likely need to take a couple of additional days off from work.

Discomfort

Because your eyes are numb during surgery, you will feel no pain during either LASIK or PRK. Mild to moderate discomfort is typical with PRK during the first twenty-four to forty-eight hours after surgery. The discomfort is caused by the absence of the epithelium, and disappears as the new epithelium grows over the area of laser treatment. In LASIK, the epithelium is not removed, so post-operative pain is usually minimal and lasts only about two to four hours.

Medications

Postoperative medications also vary between the procedures. PRK patients may use medicated eyedrops for anywhere from 1 week to three months after surgery. LASIK patients, on the other hand, are typically finished with their medications within a week after surgery.

Final Vision

The final visual results achieved by LASIK and PRK are the same, although it takes longer for the eye to heal completely with PRK. You achieve your final vision in PRK in one to three months, whereas with LASIK this typically occurs in two to four weeks.

Questions to Ask Your Surgeon about PRK

- What results can I expect?
- How long will the correction last?
- What about risks and complications?
- When can I go back to work?

- Will I need enhancement surgery?
- If I have dry eyes, will it affect my PRK surgery?
- If I've had previous eye surgeries, am I still a candidate for PRK?
- Can I wear contact lenses after surgery, if necessary?
- Could the surgery cause problems years from now?

Variations on PRK: LASEK and Epi-LASIK

You may have heard of two other laser procedures—LASEK and epi-LASIK. These procedures are very similar to PRK. The only difference is the technical method by which the surgeon removes the epithelium, the surface layer of clear skin that covers the eye. In PRK, the cells are removed by the laser, an automated brush, or gentle debridement. In LASEK, the cells are removed by loosening them with an alcohol solution. In epi-LASIK, an automated machine is used that peels off the cell layer. The results of PRK, LASEK, and epi-LASIK are identical, as are the risks and recovery time. From a patient's perspective, LASEK and epi-LASIK are indistinguishable from PRK.

10

LASIK and PRK Statistics: Your Chances for Success

W hat are my chances of achieving 20/20 vision with LASIK or PRK? This is what every patient wants to know. A better question might be this: What is the likelihood that my procedure will be successful, given my refractive error? Although it would be unreasonable to be guaranteed 20/20 eyesight after vision correction surgery, it is reasonable for you to ask your doctor to predict your chances for a successful outcome.

If you have chosen an experienced surgeon—someone who has performed 3,000 LASIK procedures at the absolute minimum—he or she has most likely performed surgery on a number of patients with vision like yours. Accordingly, you will be able to get an idea of what you can reasonably expect after LASIK or PRK.

The Importance of Statistics

Fortunately, now that the LASIK and PRK procedures have been around for several years, outcomes can be predicted by using scientific data. Each surgeon achieves somewhat different results with the same procedure. The best surgeons track their own results and adjust the laser to optimize each patient's outcome based on the surgeon's personal results. It takes about 3,000 surgeries for a surgeon to develop statistics for his or her results. If you have found a surgeon who tracks outcomes and compiles statistics based on 3,000 or more LASIK procedures, so much the better. The reality is that most surgeons have not compiled personal statistics, for one of three reasons: first, they haven't done enough procedures; second, they aren't willing to do the labor-intensive work of entering large numbers of cases into a database; or third, they don't have the statistical knowledge necessary to analyze their results. This is unfortunate, because it reduces patients' chances of achieving a perfect 20/20 result.

A surgeon who tracks his own results can give you a better result and can also better educate you about what result you can expect if you choose him or her as your surgeon. Statistics and percentages are useful to patients who want to know what kind of vision they can realistically expect after surgery. But these statistics can also be confusing or misleading. For example, when a surgeon talks about the percentage of LASIK patients who achieved 20/20 vision, this might include all patients. Or it might be limited to those patients who had only the initial LASIK procedure (no enhancements). Meanwhile, other surgeons prefer to use 20/40 as the baseline. Since patients will find inconsistencies from center to center on how this information is presented, it is crucial to pay attention to what the numbers are really telling you.

The Statistics to Know

What are the important statistics for you as a patient to know, and how can you interpret outcomes? You likely want to know your chances of achieving at least 20/40 vision. This is a key number, because 20/40 vision is required to drive legally without eyeglasses or contacts. You will also want to know your chances of achieving optimal 20/20 vision.

All of the above numbers will vary according to the surgeon you choose and your prescription. For example, patients with higher degrees of nearsightedness, farsightedness, or astigmatism are more likely to need an enhancement procedure.

Statistical Outcomes According to Your Refraction

As you have learned in this book, LASIK and PRK are very similar, and the same laser is used for both procedures. So it shouldn't surprise you that the statistics are the same for PRK and LASIK: your chance of getting 20/20 vision doesn't depend on which procedure you choose. The decision of whether to have LASIK or PRK is based on other factors—which procedure is safer for your eye and which gives you the better recovery.

Your chance of achieving 20/20 vision depends on how nearsighted or farsighted you are. To use this chapter, find your most recent eyeglass or contact lens prescription and look at the first number for each eye (see "Understanding your Eyeglass Prescription" in chapter 1). This is the sphere part of the prescription. The statistics listed below, based on the sphere, give you an indication of the results to expect from wavefront-guided laser treatment by an experienced surgeon. Keep in mind that the patients in these statistics who did not achieve 20/20 vision without correction are usually still pleased with their results. They can do most things without eyeglasses or contacts, including driving a car. And when it is absolutely necessary for them to fine-tune their vision, they can still wear eyeglasses.

Myopia
Mild Myopia

You have mild nearsightedness if the sphere part of your eyeglass prescription is between 0.00 and minus 3.00 (negative 3.00) diopters.

A patient with mild nearsightedness, or myopia, has essentially a 100 percent chance of achieving 20/40 vision or better and being able to drive without eyeglasses or contacts. The chance of achieving 20/20 vision on the first procedure is higher than 95 percent, and if enhancements are included, it rises to above 99 percent.

Moderate Myopia

You have moderate myopia if the sphere part of your eyeglass prescription is between minus 3.00 and minus 7.00 diopters. After the initial procedure, 99 percent of patients with moderate myopia achieve 20/40 vision or better. Of these, more than 90 percent achieve 20/20 vision or better. Including enhancement surgery, 100 percent of patients see 20/40 or better, and 99 percent see 20/20 or better.

A common misconception among patients in their late 40s and mid-50s is that they'll have perfect vision—far and near—after LASIK. They will need glasses for small print, unless they receive monovision—one eye corrected for distance and one for close up vision.

High Myopia

You have high myopia if the sphere part of your eyeglass prescription is between minus 7.00 and minus 10.00 diopters. Patients with high myopia have a 98 percent chance of seeing 20/40 or better after the initial procedure and an 85 percent change of seeing 20/20. Including enhancement surgeries, they have a greater than 99 percent chance of seeing 20/40 or better and a 95 percent chance of seeing 20/20 or better.

Extreme Myopia

If the sphere part of your eyeglass prescription is more than minus 11.00, you have extreme myopia. Patients with extreme myopia have a 94 percent chance of achieving 20/40 vision or better after the initial procedure. Including enhancements, 90 percent of patients will have 20/20 vision or better.

Many patients with extreme myopia do well with LASIK, but we do not consider them optimal candidates. After LASIK patients in this range are more likely to have enhancements and more likely to have problems with quality of vision, such as glare, halos, or hazy vision. Patients in this group need to thoroughly discuss the risks and benefits of LASIK, as well as other options, with their doctors. Although enhancement rates are higher in this group of patients, because of other variables in the eye, there may be limitations on what can be done. Most surgeons do not generally recommend PRK for these patients, who may be better candidates for the implantable contact lens (see chapter 11, "Other Vision Correction Procedures").

Hyperopia
Low and Moderate Hyperopia

If the sphere part of your eyeglass prescription is a positive number, you have farsightedness, or hyperopia. If the number is between 0.00 and +4.00, you have a low to moderate level of hyperopia. After your initial LASIK or PRK procedure, you have a 95 percent chance of achieving 20/40 vision or better and a 75 percent chance of achieving 20/20 vision.

Patients treated for hyperopia should be aware that their healing time will be slightly longer than for patients with myopia, and the chance that they will need an enhancement is slightly higher. These numbers will vary according to the patient's original prescription and the skill and experience level of the surgeon.

High Hyperopia

If the sphere part of your eyeglass prescription is more than +4.00, you have a high degree of hyperopia. LASIK still can correct your vision up to +6.00 diopters, but the results are less predictable, and quality of vision may not be as good as for lower degrees of hyperopia. Above +6.00 diopters, LASIK is not an option for you. If you are in this range of hyperopia, you may wish to consider refractive lens exchange or an implantable contact lens. See chapter 11 for more details.

Astigmatism

Astigmatism is the second number on your eyeglass prescription for each eye. Patients with mild astigmatism (less than 1.00) can expect outcomes and enhancement percentages nearly identical to those patients with myopia or hyperopia only. The presence of a greater degree of preoperative astigmatism will somewhat reduce your chance of achieving 20/20 vision after the initial procedure, making it more likely that you will want to have an enhancement. Astigmatism of 6 diopters or less can be corrected with either LASIK or PRK.

11

Other Vision-Correction Procedures

If it turns out that you are not a good candidate for LASIK or PRK, you and your eye doctor may wish to consider other surgical options. One of the procedures described here may be appropriate.

Intacs Corneal Ring Segments

Insertion of *Intacs corneal ring segments* was formerly offered to patients with mild myopia and minimal astigmatism as another option for correcting their nearsightedness. Small, thin arcs of plastic are inserted into the peripheral part of the cornea. Each arc looks like a half circle. These ring segments reshape the eye, correcting mild levels of nearsightedness. Intacs corneal ring segments are no longer used to correct myopia, because the results are less accurate than LASIK and the ring segments cannot correct astigmatism. Today, the ring segments are primarily used to treat keratoconus and ectasia.

Astigmatic Keratotomy

Astigmatic keratotomy (AK) corrects only astigmatism. Usually, one or two incisions are made in the peripheral cornea to make it rounder (as if loosening the laces on a football). This procedure has a long track record but is rarely used today by itself, because it is significantly less accurate than PRK and LASIK for correcting astigmatism.

The most frequent use of AK today is for the correction of astigmatism at the time of lens implant surgery (either cataract or refractive lens exchange surgery). AK also goes by the name "relaxing incisions."

Lens Surgery
Cataract Surgery

For patients with significant cataracts who are looking to correct their nearsightedness or farsightedness, *cataract surgery* presents the best option. A cataract is a haziness of the natural lens inside the eye that impairs vision. After removing the cataract, the surgeon can implant a lens that will reduce or eliminate nearsightedness and farsightedness and potentially reduce presbyopia. Astigmatism, too, can be treated at the time of cataract surgery, either with AK (see above) or with a special astigmatic lens implant.

Modern cataract surgery, when performed by an experienced surgeon, can allow patients a recovery period rather similar to that of LASIK. In its most sophisticated form, cataract surgery can be performed with eyedrop anesthesia (as with LASIK or PRK) and require no sutures. An outpatient procedure in skilled hands, it takes twenty minutes or less to complete.

Refractive Lens Exchange

Refractive lens exchange (RLE) involves removing the eye's natural lens, as in a cataract operation. A flexible synthetic lens implant is then placed inside the eye through a tiny incision to correct nearsightedness or farsightness. RLE is a painless outpatient procedure. The tiny incision closes by itself, without sutures. Visual recovery is quite rapid. As with LASIK, most patients are able to return to work the day after their procedure.

RLE is most commonly performed to treat higher levels of near-sightedness or farsightedness in patients over age forty. The optical results are superior to LASIK for these higher corrections. RLE may also be fine-tuned with LASIK if a small refractive error remains. Some surgeons use RLE to treat extremely nearsighted or farsighted patients who are not candidates for LASIK or PRK.

The major drawbacks of RLE are the risk of *postoperative retinal detachment* (more of a risk with nearsighted than farsighted patients) and the risks that accompany any intraocular surgery, including the extremely rare chance of an infection in the eye.

If both eyes are corrected for distance vision, RLE patients will require reading glasses after their procedure. As with LASIK and PRK, however, monovision corrections are possible with RLE to decrease or even eliminate one's need for reading glasses. Or new intraocular lenses, called *presbyopic lenses*, can be implanted at the time of lens extraction. These lenses allow a patient to see both near and far after the operation. For the best results, both eyes should be implanted with the multifocal lens. Certain lens designs may cause some patients to experience a loss of contrast at night and also develop halos around lights. If these symptoms become problematic, the lens can be removed and replaced with a conventional lens implant.

RLE is generally not performed on younger patients, because the surgery involves removing the natural lens, which in young people allows them to read without glasses. Either LASIK or *contact lens implants* is usually a better option for younger patients, because these procedures preserve reading vision.

Conductive Keratoplasty

With *conductive keratoplasty* (CK), a special probe introduces an electrical current to the peripheral cornea, shrinking the corneal fibers.

The effect is like the tightening of a belt, and the central cornea steepens. With CK, only one eye is treated. The procedure is primarily used to make the one treated eye nearsighted to create good reading vision in people over age forty-five who have excellent distance vision. The procedure takes less than five minutes and is painless. The major advantage of CK is its relative safety. Because no tissue is removed and all the work is done on the peripheral cornea, the risk of impairment of vision is slight.

Candidates for CK for the correction of presbyopia (improvement of reading vision) should be at least forty-five years old and have good distance vision. Recovery of reading vision is immediate. Distance vision in the treated eye is reduced somewhat. The major disadvantage of CK is that the results may not be permanent. After two to three years, either the treatment is repeated or the patient can have a permanent LASIK correction.

Contact Lens Implants

A *contact lens implant* may correct either extreme nearsightedness or extreme farsightedness. Unlike with cataract surgery, the natural lens is not removed; rather, the implant sits in front of the natural lens. In effect, the contact lens implant becomes an internal contact lens.

Implantable contact lens technology has arisen out of the advances in modern cataract surgery. Current technology allows ophthalmologists to insert flexible *intraocular lenses* (used to replace the natural lens after cataract surgery) through extremely small incisions. Some contact lens implants, too, are flexible enough to allow folding as they are inserted through small incision openings.

Because of the slightly increased risk of more serious complications, contact lens implants are reserved for high amounts of nearsightedness or farsightedness—beyond the safe limits of LASIK. These lenses are typically reserved for patients with myopia greater than 9 to 10 diopters and hyperopia greater than 4 diopters. In addition, contact lens implants may be preferable to LASIK in patients who fall within the safe LASIK parameters with regard to their prescription but who have thinner corneas, making the tissue-removal aspect of LASIK less desirable. These lenses are implanted one eye at a time in an outpatient procedure that takes ten to twenty-five minutes.

Implantable contact lenses are very safe. Risks unique to contact lens implants include causing a cataract, damage to the inner layer of the cornea, or an infection in the eye. Such complications are very rare. In large FDA studies of these lenses with thousands of patients treated, no patient lost vision from these lenses. Other risks are similar to those of LASIK and PRK: undercorrection, overcorrection, and nighttime glare. Undercorrections and overcorrections can often be treated with a LASIK enhancement, because the remaining correction is usually very small.

Advantages of the implantable contact lenses include a more accurate correction and better night vision than with LASIK or PRK. Also, these lenses are removable if for any reason a patient is unsatisfied with his or her vision. After the implants are removed, vision returns to where it was before surgery.

Relatively few surgeons today have the experience to implant these lenses, but more and more surgeons are learning the procedure. We expect it to become widely available in the next five to ten years.

Bioptics

Bioptics is a combination procedure involving a contact lens implant followed by LASIK. It is recommended for the most extreme levels of myopia and hyperopia (with or without astigmatism) when neither technique alone will entirely correct the refractive error. This combined technique can be used to correct over 30.00 diopters of myopia—nearly three times the maximum that can be safely corrected with LASIK.

Surgery for Presbyopia

One of the more exciting areas of ophthalmology is the surgical treatment of presbyopia—the stiffening of the natural lens that decreases near vision as we age. A number of new devices are under investigation, including replacement lenses that are intended to flex like the natural lens and methods of strengthening the muscles that pull on the lens. To date, all of these devices have problems and limitations, but the problems are being slowly addressed. It is likely that, in the next ten to fifteen years, a good treatment for presbyopia will be available. Having LASIK now will not disqualify you from having these treatments in the future.

Closing Remarks

LASIK vision correction is the most popular refractive surgery performed today. Its reputation is well deserved, as people discover that LASIK delivers good vision safely when it is performed by experienced, skilled surgeons. Perhaps more telling than the general public's enthusiasm for LASIK, however, is the widespread acceptance the procedure has gained among professionals in the fields of ophthalmology and optometry. In fact, more eye doctors have had LASIK on their own eyes than any other group of people.

What does the future hold for people who could benefit from laser vision correction? Currently in the United States, myopia, hyperopia, and astigmatism have all been approved for treatment, but only for refractive errors that fall within certain parameters. Newer laser technology is being developed that expands these parameters; this will make it possible to treat patients with more severe vision problems in the future.

The issue of gradually losing one's near vision after age forty, or presbyopia, still looms. A number of medical research efforts are now under way to develop procedures that could restore near vision in the vast majority of aging patients. Some of the research involves new techniques to reshape the cornea; others, to restore the function of the focusing muscles of the eye; and still others, that concentrate on the lens itself.

Newer lasers now entering the marketplace offer customizable programs that allow surgeons to treat patients with irregular corneas on a patient-by-patient basis.

Finally, there are new tracking devices that lock the excimer laser beam onto the patient's eye. If the patient's eye moves, the laser moves with it. This innovation should benefit patients who find it difficult to fix their eyes in one place and those who require particularly long treatments.

In its current state, LASIK has proven to be a life-changing experience for many. However, the decision to have LASIK is an important one that ultimately only you can make. We hope to have given you information that will help you make sound decisions based on facts, not on hopes or misconceptions.

Resources

International Society of Refractive Surgery of the American Academy of Ophthalmology (ISRS/AAO)
PO Box 7424
San Francisco, CA 94120-7424
Phone: (415) 561-8500
www.isrs.org
www.aao.org

The International Society of Refractive Surgery of the American Academy of Ophthalmology (ISRS/AAO) is an international organization of eye-care professionals dedicated to refractive surgery. ISRS/AAO was formed in 2003 when the International Society of Refractive Surgery (ISRS) and the American Academy of Ophthalmology's Refractive Surgery Interest Group (RSIG) joined forces. ISRS/AAO offers courses, scientific journals, and other educational and professional services to eye doctors. Of interest to consumers are the "Locate an ISRS Doctor" and "Find an Eye MD" search engines located on each Web site. Both list refractive surgeons and board-certified ophthalmologists who specialize in refractive surgery.

American Society of Cataract and Refractive Surgery (ASCRS)
4000 Legato Road, Suite 850
Fairfax, VA 22033
Phone: (703) 591-2220
www.ascrs.org

The American Society of Cataract and Refractive Surgery (ASCRS) is an international educational and scientific organization whose 8,000 member ophthalmologists specialize in cataract and refractive surgery. ASCRS members are recognized leaders and innovators in ophthalmic surgery worldwide. This site is geared toward physicians, but it also offers helpful consumer eye-care information. The "Find a Surgeon" feature provides a list of ASCRS member eye surgeons by zip code.

Eye Surgery Education Council
750 Washington Street, Box 450
Boston, MA 02111
Phone: (617) 636-5754
www.lasikinstitute.org

This Eye Surgery Education Council organization is a nonprofit educational organization dedicated to promoting the best possible understanding and practice of LASIK. The site provides comprehensive, consumer-friendly information about LASIK surgery.

National Eye Institute (NEI)
31 Center Drive
MSC 2510
Bethesda, MD 20892-3655
Phone: (301) 496-5248
www.nei.nih.gov

The National Eye Institute (NEI) supports more than 80 percent of the vision research conducted in the United States at approximately 250 medical centers, hospitals, universities, and other institutions. In addition, the Institute conducts studies in its own facilities in Bethesda, Maryland, to combat the myriad eye disorders affecting millions of people worldwide. The site lists current NEI-supported clinical trials and how to participate in them and includes an online fact sheet for finding eye-care professionals and a fact sheet on how to obtain financial aid for eye care. NEI also offers free publications that can be ordered online.

American Board of Medical Specialties (ABMS)

1007 Church Street, Suite 404
Evanston, IL 60201-5913
Phone Verification on surgeons: (866) ASK-ABMS
Phone: (847) 491-9091
www.abms.org

The American Board of Medical Specialties (ABMS) is the umbrella organization for the twenty-four approved medical specialty boards in the United States. Established in 1933, the ABMS serves to coordinate the activities of its member boards and to provide information to the public, the government, the profession, and its members concerning issues involving specialization and certification in medicine. The mission of the ABMS is to maintain and improve the quality of medical care in the United States by assisting the member boards in their efforts to develop and utilize professional and educational standards for the evaluation and certification of physician specialists.

Federation of State Medical Boards

Federation Place
400 Fuller Wiser Road, Suite 300
Euless, TX 76039-3855
Phone: (817) 868-4000
www.fsmb.org

The Federation of State Medical Boards of the United States, Inc., is a national organization comprising the sixty-nine medical boards of the United States, the District of Columbia, Puerto Rico, Guam, and the U.S. Virgin Islands. The mission is to be a leader in improving the quality, safety, and integrity of health care in the United States by promoting high standards for physician licensure and practice. FSMB operates the Federation Physician Data Center, a nationally recognized system for collecting, recording, and distributing to state medical boards and other appropriate agencies data on disciplinary actions taken against licensees by the boards and other governmental authorities.

Food and Drug Administration

5600 Fishers Lane (HFE-88)
Rockville, MD 20852
www.fda.gov

The U.S. Food and Drug Administration (FDA), which oversees the safety of food, cosmetics, medicines, medical devices, and radiation-emitting products, also has a consumer-friendly Web site. An entire section devoted to LASIK includes educational articles written for the layperson. Also posted are consumer updates, a list of FDA-approved lasers, a directory for consumer and manufacturer calls and complaints, and links to other online FDA manuals and publications. Detailed information about the results of FDA authorized studies are posted on the Web site.

U.S. National Library of Medicine
8600 Rockville Pike
Bethesda, MD 20894
Phone: 888-FIND-NLM, 888-346-3656; 301-594-5983
www.nlm.nih.gov/medlineplus

Designed primarily for health professionals and scientists, the National Library of Medicine Web site, called MedlinePlus, is a collection of authoritative health information drawn from the National Library of Medicine, the National Institutes of Health, and other government agencies and health-related organizations. The site offers up-to-date health news, an illustrated medical encyclopedia, a medical dictionary, and interactive patient tutorials. Users can view articles on health-related topics from more than 3,500 medical journals and can search through more than 650 topics, including laser eye surgery.

HealthFinder
www.healthfinder.gov

HealthFinder is a service of the U.S. Department of Health and Human Services. Written for the consumer, the Web site features articles on timely health topics, the latest government health news, advice and how-to tips for patients, links to online journals, and links to medical databases. The site also posts LASIK-related Web resources through keyword search.

Glossary

Ablate: To remove, or vaporize, tissue, using laser energy.

Ablation zone: The area of tissue removed by the laser. Also called the treatment zone.

Accommodation: The ability of the eye's lens to fine-tune focus by flexing—becoming more or less convex—as needed. Accommodation can compensate for minor focusing problems in younger people whose lens and surrounding muscles are still limber and pliable.

All laser LASIK: This term has been used to describe both the Intralase microkeratome and PRK.

Anterior ciliary sclerotomy (ACS): A surgical procedure intended to relieve presbyopia. Several small incisions are made in the sclera (white part of the eye) directly over the muscle that controls the lens. The results of the procedure are poor, and very few doctors perform it.

Antibiotic drops: Eyedrops containing medicine that prevents infection by killing or inhibiting harmful bacteria.

Anti-inflammatory drops: Eyedrops containing medicine that counteracts inflammation, usually a steroid or a nonsteroidal medicine similar to ibuprofin.

Artificial tears: Sterile eyedrops used to lubricate the eyes the same way natural tears do.

Astigmatism: A refractive error caused by an asymmetrically shaped cornea. Rather than being round in shape like a basketball, an astigmatic cornea is shaped like a football, causing light to come to several points of focus instead of meeting at a single point of focus. People with astigmatism experience blurred images or double vision.

Automated lamellar keratoplasty (ALK): An older refractive surgery, developed in 1987, in which the surgeon first creates an extremely thin flap in the uppermost layer of the cornea, using a device called a microkeratome, and then makes a second pass with the microkeratome to remove additional tissue. It is not performed anymore.

Axis: A measurement of the direction of astigmatism. The astigmatic cornea is oval in shape, and axis is the angle of the long direction of the oval with a horizontal line.

Benchmarking: The process of tracking statistical outcomes for the purpose of predicting future outcomes. With LASIK, statistics from 1,000 or more procedures can provide a good basis for benchmarking.

Best corrected vision: The best possible vision achieved with corrective eyeglass lenses.

Blended vision: See monovision.

Board certified: A credential awarded to physicians who have undergone the additional training and proved proficiency in an area by passing a rigorous examination. Ninety percent of ophthalmologists are board certified, so this credential is of limited value in distinguishing one ophthalmologist from another. If a surgeon is not board certified in ophthalmology, beware!

Cataract: Clouding of the natural lens within the eye, causing blurry vision.

Central island: A treatable complication from LASIK in which a small, raised area in the center of the cornea's treatment zone results from its having received less laser energy than the surrounding tissue. Central islands can cause distorted vision.

Comanagement: An arrangement in which the surgeon does the surgery and the primary eye doctor does all or part of the preoperative or postoperative care. Ideally comanagement offers the advantage of a second expert to oversee care and ensure the patient's satisfaction with the results.

Constrict: To become smaller.

Cornea: The outer, dome-shaped, transparent part of the eye that bulges out at the front of the eyeball and covers the iris and pupil. Its curvature causes light to bend. The cornea provides most of the eye's focusing power. It is the only part of the eye on which LASIK is performed.

Corneal topographer: An instrument that creates a three-dimensional map of the cornea, using computerized analysis.

Crystalline lens: See lens.

Cylinder: One of three measures in an eyeglass prescription. It indicates whether astigmatism is present, and to what degree.

Diffuse lamellar keratitis (DLK): A potential complication of LASIK; also known as "sands of the Sahara" syndrome. DLK is a noninfectious inflammation that arises between the corneal flap and the underlying stroma.

Dilate: To become larger, as when the pupil enlarges in very dim light conditions.

Diopter: A measurement of how strong a lens is. Thicker lenses have a higher number of diopters. In eye care, it is used to measure your refractive error, or what eyeglass lens is needed to correct your vision. Hyperopia is measured in terms of positive diopters. Myopia is measured in terms of negative diopters.

Disease neutral: Something that neither prevents diseases nor affects the treatment of diseases. LASIK is considered disease neutral.

Dry eye: A condition characterized by corneal dryness due to inadequate tear production.

Endothelium: The innermost layer of the cornea, a single cell thick, that helps regulate the cornea's hydration.

Enhancement procedure: A secondary treatment with the excimer laser to fine-tune one's visual acuity after the initial LASIK procedure. Enhancements take place after vision has stabilized, usually three to six months after LASIK. Enhancements usually do not require making a new corneal flap.

Epithelial ingrowth: A potential complication of LASIK produced when corneal surface cells, or epithelium, grow underneath the corneal flap during the first month after surgery. The condition is often easily diagnosed and treated.

Epi-LASIK: A variant of PRK in which the epithelium (the clear skin that covers the eye) is peeled off by an automated machine called an epikeratome. The results are the same with PRK.

Epithelium: The thin, protective outermost surface of the cornea. It is made up of the same kind of cells that cover

most of the body. The epithelium grows rapidly, and continually regenerates.

Excimer laser: The type of laser used in refractive surgery to
remove corneal tissue. It emits highly precise pulses of ultraviolet light to break up tissue one molecular layer at a time,
vaporizing it without generating heat that could damage surrounding tissue.

Eyelid speculum: A device placed between the upper and lower
eyelids to keep the patient from blinking during surgery. It is
painless, because the eye is anesthetized.

Farsightedness: See hyperopia.

Food and Drug Administration (FDA): The federal agency that
regulates the manufacturers and distributors of drugs and
devices. There is a popular misconception that the FDA regulates the practice of medicine. It does not; regulation of the
practice of medicine is left up to the states. A related misconception is that the FDA approves medical and surgical procedures. It does not—the majority of medical and surgical
procedures done in the United States are not FDA-approved
but rather are off-label, or unapproved.

Ghosting: The appearance of double images or shadows around
images. Ghosting is sometimes experienced by people with
astigmatism and can also result from irregular healing of the
corneal surface after LASIK.

Glaucoma: A disorder of the eye characterized by an increase of
pressure within the eyeball.

Halo: A complication of LASIK in which the patient sees a glow
around lights at night. Halos usually decrease over time.

Haze: Scarring of the corneal stroma, or corneal bed. Significant haze occurs rarely after PRK, and does not occur after LASIK.

Herpes simplex: A recurrent viral infection of the eye characterized by a painful sore on the eyelid or surface of the eye. It causes inflammation of the cornea and can lead to blindness. This is not a sexually transmitted infection. Patients with herpes simplex of the eye may not be candidates for LASIK.

Higher-order aberration: Irregularity of vision that cannot be corrected by glasses or contact lenses.

Hyperopia: Also known as farsightedness, hyperopia occurs when the eyeball is too short from front to back or when the eye's focusing mechanism is too weak, causing light rays to be focused behind, rather than on, the retina. People with hyperopia see objects at a distance more clearly than close up but usually have difficulty with both distance and near vision.

Induced astigmatism: A rare complication of LASIK in which astigmatism develops after the initial surgery. Most people can tolerate a small degree of astigmatism. In more serious cases, induced astigmatism can be treated with an enhancement, if necessary.

Inflammation: A localized response to an injury that results in redness, heat, pain, and swelling and that can result in tissue damage if left untreated.

Informed consent: A legal form a patient is asked to sign that thoroughly discusses the risks, benefits, alternative options, and possible complications of LASIK.

IntraLase: A laser-based microkeratome that helps the surgeon create the flap by creating thousands of tiny explosions in the cornea. The surgeon then dissects the flap free with a blunt separator. Some surgeons prefer the Intralase microkeratome, while others prefer the newer automated microkeratomes that do not require manual dissection of the flap.

Intraocular pressure: The pressure exerted by the fluid within the eye that gives it its firmness and round shape.

Iris: The colored ring of tissue in the eye that is behind the cornea and in front of the lens. The muscles of the iris can adjust the size of the eye's opening, or pupil, to allow for larger or smaller amounts of light to enter the eye.

Keratectomy: Surgical removal of any part of the cornea. In the context of LASIK, keratectomy is the flap-making part of the procedure.

Keratomileusis: Any process of carving, or reshaping, the cornea.

Lamellar: An adjective meaning "layered." Lamellar corneal surgery corrects focusing errors by removing or reshaping some of the corneal layers.

Laser thermal keratoplasty (LTK): A technique that uses heat energy to change the shape of the cornea and that is designed to correct only low amounts of farsightedness. A special laser is used to deliver laser energy to the peripheral cornea to slightly tighten the fibers and thereby steepen its curvature. The LTK procedure may also be useful for treating occasional overcorrections from LASIK procedures. It is similar to conductive keratoplasty (see chapter 11) but has largely been abandoned, because it was found that the effect wore off too quickly.

LASEK: A variant of PRK in which the epithelium (the clear skin that covers the eye) is removed by loosening it with an alcohol solution. The results are the same as those of PRK.

LASIK: An acronym for laser in-situ keratomileusis. In LASIK, a miniature automated instrument called a microkeratome creates an extremely thin, hinged flap on the surface of the cornea. After the flap is gently lifted back, the surgeon reshapes the corneal stroma, using an excimer laser. The corneal flap is then replaced, and it quickly adheres. LASIK is a safe and pain-free form of refractive eye surgery that has proven to be highly successful and popular.

Lens: The globe-shaped natural lens of the eye, located behind the iris, that helps fine-tune the angle of light to bring it to a point of focus on the retina. As the lens becomes less flexible with age, its ability to adapt its focus for reading gradually decreases.

Microkeratome: The instrument a surgeon uses to create the corneal flap in the uppermost layer of the cornea during the LASIK procedure.

Monovision: A process by which a surgeon corrects one eye for seeing at a distance and the other eye for seeing objects close up.

Myopia: Also known as nearsightedness, myopia is due to a cornea that has too much curvature or to an eyeball that is too long, causing light to be focused in front of, rather than on, the retina. People with myopia have difficulty seeing objects at a distance.

Nearsightedness: See myopia.

Nomogram: The surgeon's formula that is entered into the laser's computer calculation to further refine the manufacturer's recommended settings.

Nonfreeze keratomileusis: The process of reshaping the corneal disc directly on the eye without having to remove the disc and freeze it for the purpose of reshaping, as was done in early lamellar surgeries, precursors to LASIK.

Ophthalmology: The field of medicine dealing with diseases and conditions of the eye.

Ophthalmologist: A medical doctor specializing in the diagnosis and medical or surgical treatment of eye diseases.

Optic nerve: A bundle of nerve fibers, about the diameter of a pencil, that connect to the nerve fiber layer of the retina and terminate in the brain. The optic nerve carries the visual messages from the photoreceptors of the retina to the brain, where images are created and processed.

Optometrist: An eye-care professional specializing in the examination, diagnosis, treatment, management, and prevention of diseases and disorders of the eye. Optometrists do not perform surgery, but otherwise perform many of the functions that ophthalmologists do. Optometrists are often general eye-care providers and can provide preoperative and postoperative care for LASIK patients and other refractive surgery patients.

Orthokeratology: A technique for treating myopia by using a series of rigid contact lenses to reshape the cornea. The lenses apply pressure to the sides of the cornea, flattening them. This technique is effective for low levels of nearsightedness, but retainer contact lenses must be worn every day to prevent the effect from wearing off.

Overcorrection: A complication of LASIK, overcorrection results when the amount of correction resulting from the LASIK procedure is more than intended.

Peripheral vision: The ability to see objects and movement outside of, or on the periphery of, one's direct line of vision.

Photoablation: The process of removing, or vaporizing, tissue by means of laser energy.

Photorefractive keratectomy (PRK): A type of laser vision correction that reshapes the cornea by ablating, or vaporizing, the corneal tissue one microscopic layer at a time, using an excimer laser. Unlike with LASIK, in which a hinged corneal flap is first made and lifted back to expose the corneal bed, with PRK the sculpting process removes the outer (epithelial) layer of the cornea as the laser energy works its way down to the corneal bed.

Presbyopia: Often confused with farsightedness, presbyopia (literally, "old eyes") is the age-dependent need for reading glasses or bifocals, caused by the decreasing ability of the eye's lens and surrounding muscles to fine-tune focus.

Prescription: A series of numbers that instruct someone how to provide a patient with the proper eyeglass or contact lens (see also refractive error).

Punctum plugs: Used in the treatment of dry eye, these tiny silicone plugs are inserted into the tear-drainage openings of the eyelid to delay the drainage of natural tears so the eyes will stay moist.

Pupil: The small black dot, or opening, in the center of the iris. The pupil changes its diameter in response to changes in lighting.

Radial keratotomy (RK): A form of refractive surgery in which the surgeon alters the shape of the cornea by making thin incisions around it in a spokelike pattern. The incisions cause the central portion of the cornea to flatten, treating myopia and astigmatism. RK is not performed anymore.

Refract: To bend, as when light passes through a curved shape such as a cornea or lens.

Refraction: The art of measuring the refractive error of the eye. Also, a synonym for refractive error.

Refractive error: The eyeglass prescription needed to correct your vision. Refractive error has three parts: sphere (how nearsighted or farsighted you are), cylinder (how much astigmatism you have), and axis (the angle of your astigmatism).

Refractive surgery: Any type of surgery that changes the focusing power of the eye in order to correct a refractive error. LASIK is a type of refractive surgery that corrects the eye's focusing ability by reshaping the curvature of the cornea.

Regression: A potential complication of LASIK in which the vision tends to drift back, or regress, toward its original refractive error.

Retina: The light-sensitive layer of cells on the inner back surface of the eye that processes light and functions much like film in a camera. The retina converts light into electrical impulses, which are transmitted along the optic nerve to the brain, which in turn interprets the impulses as images.

Sclera: The tough "white" of the eye that makes up five-sixths of the outer layer of the eyeball. Along with the cornea, it protects the eyeball.

Scleral expansion bands (SEBs): Used in surgical reversal of presbyopia, these thin silicon bands are implanted in the sclera to expand the equator of the eye, ostensibly to restore accommodation and relieve presbyopia. The theory behind SEB is that expansion of the eye will allow increased room for the lens to move normally, enabling the eye to see nearby objects again. A number of studies now suggest that this procedure is ineffective.

Snellen eye chart: The standard eye chart used by eye doctors to determine visual acuity.

Sphere: One of three measurements taken during an eye examination to arrive at one's eyeglass prescription. The sphere measures where the eye focuses light—on the retina (normal vision), in front of the retina (myopia), or behind the retina (hyperopia).

Starburst: A visual aberration in which the patient sees rays radiating from lights viewed at night. Starbursts may be seen by people who wear eyeglasses and contact lenses, and are sometimes experienced by patients who have undergone LASIK.

Striae: Wrinkles or folds in the corneal flap that are a potential complication of LASIK. Small striae, call microstriae, usually do not affect vision. Larger striae, or macrostriae, can be smoothed out easily.

Stroma: The strong, fibrous layer that makes up 90 percent of the cornea's thickness and provides the cornea with its structure and shape. Also called the stromal bed, this is the part of the cornea sculpted with the laser in LASIK surgery.

Surgical reversal of presbyopia (SRP): See scleral expansion bands.

Tonometry: The measure of intraocular pressure, or the pressure inside the eye.

Topical corticosteroid: A medicated eyedrop that prevents inflammation of the eye tissue after LASIK surgery.

Undercorrection: A complication of LASIK; results when the amount of correction resulting from the LASIK procedure is less than intended. Most undercorrections can be treated with an enhancement procedure.

Visual acuity: The sharpness or clarity of vision that enables one to distinguish fine details and shapes.

Vitreous humor: The gel-like substance, composed of about 99 percent water, that fills the main cavity of the eye between the lens and the retinal wall.

Wavefront analysis: A measurement, performed with laser light rays, of irregularities in the eyeball.

Index

About the Authors

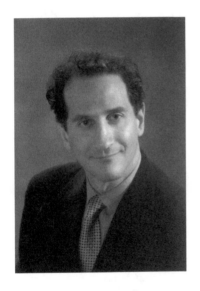

Ernest W. Kornmehl, MD, FACS, is a board-certified ophthalmologist and the medical director of the Kornmehl Laser Eye Associates, in Boston. He completed his ophthalmology residency and chief residency at the Yale Eye Center, Yale School of Medicine, followed by a Heed fellowship in corneal surgery at the Massachusetts Eye and Ear Infirmary, Harvard Medical School. He also served as director of the Novatec Laser Surgery Program for Nearsightedness at the Massachusetts Eye and Ear Infirmary, Harvard Medical School. Dr. Kornmehl is a clinical instructor at Harvard Medical School, an associate clinical professor of ophthalmology at the Tufts School of Medicine, and a research associate at the Massachusetts Institute of Technology.

Dr. Kornmehl has taught surgery for nearsightedness and astigmatism at the American Academy of Ophthalmology (AAO) since

1987. He is a recipient of the AAO Honor Award and Senior Achievement Award for his numerous scientific presentations and instruction courses, is listed as a top LASIK surgeon and ophthalmologist by *Boston* magazine's Top Doctors issue, has been selected by his peers to be listed in *Best Doctors in America*, and in Castle and Connolly's *America's Top Doctors.*

He serves as an examiner for the American Board of Ophthalmology, is a past president of the Massachusetts Society of Eye Physicians and Surgeons, and has served as president of Boston Aid to the Blind. Dr. Kornmehl has served as a member of the Patient Education Committee of the American Academy of Ophthalmology and was an appointee by the governor of Massachusetts to the Commission for the Blind.

Dr. Kornmehl is the developer of the Kornmehl LASIK System, specialized instruments used worldwide during the LASIK procedure. Dr. Kornmehl is also codeveloper of the S-K (Swinger-Kornmehl) solution, which is used to reduce corneal swelling.

Dr. Kornmehl lectures nationally and internationally, is the author of numerous scientific publications and chapters in textbooks, and serves on the editorial boards of *Ophthalmology Times* and *EyeNet*, an official publication of the AAO. He has received several research grants from the National Institutes of Health, has participated as a principal investigator in FDA clinical trials, and has developed a method of transforming skin into corneal tissue.

Dr. Kornmehl has been quoted in the *Journal of the American Medical Association, Health News/New England Journal of Medicine,* the *New York Times*, the *Wall Street Journal*, the *Boston Globe*, the *Los Angeles Times*, the *Washington Post, Vogue, Business Week, People* magazine, *Reader's Digest, Family Circle, Good Housekeeping, Mademoiselle, Prevention* magazine, *Men's Health, Fitness, More* magazine, and *USA Today*. He has been interviewed by WBZ-TV, WCVB-TV,

WB56-TV, CBS Evening News/Healthwatch, CNN, World News Tonight, and the Today show.

Dr. Kornmehl may be reached through his Web site: **www.visionboston.com**.

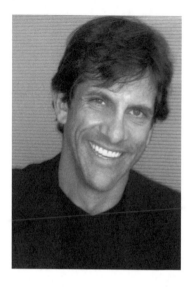

Jonathan M. Davidorf, MD, is a board-certified ophthalmologist and the director of the Davidorf Eye Group, in West Hills, California, where he specializes in laser vision correction and lens implant surgery. He is an assistant clinical professor at UCLA's Jules Stein Eye Institute and has served as director of surgeon training for Refractec, Inc., chief ophthalmologist for the Women's World Cup, and codirector of Friends of Vision Foundation, a nonprofit organization that provides medical and surgical ophthalmologic care to underdeveloped nations.

Dr. Davidorf was an Academic All-American at the University of California, Berkeley; he continued his training at the University of California, San Diego; UCLA; and Ohio State University. He completed an international fellowship in refractive surgery in South America, where he researched and helped develop LASIK and other refractive surgery techniques, several years before their approval in the United States.

Among his publications are the definitive scientific papers on implantable contact lenses and Bioptics vision-correction surgery and pioneering work on pediatric LASIK. Dr. Davidorf is also coauthor of LASIK: Principles and Techniques, the first medical textbook on LASIK. He has served as investigator for many clinical trials, including the investigations that led to FDA approval of LASIK. In 1999, Dr. Davidorf received recognition from the International Society of Refractive Surgery for best research by a vision scientist.

Dr. Davidorf has delivered award-winning presentations to national and international audiences on the subject of refractive surgery and continues to train other ophthalmologists on advanced surgical techniques. His course Emerging Technologies in Cataract and Refractive Surgery is attended by surgeons from around the world. He is a lecturer and course director for the American Academy of Ophthalmology, the American Society of Cataract and Refractive Surgery, and the International Society of Refractive Surgery. For his contributions, Dr. Davidorf received the American Academy of Ophthalmology's Achievement Award, and was a Guest of Honor at their Annual Meeting in 2005.

Dr. Davidorf received Bausch & Lomb's Clarity Award in 2003 for his leadership of and experience with wavefront technology and in 2004 was selected as one of America's top ophthalmologists by the Consumers' Research Council of America. His media appearances include news telecasts for ABC, CBS, NBC, and Fox. He has also been interviewed for numerous radio programs and has been featured in newspaper and magazine articles coast to coast.

Dr. Davidorf may be reached at the Davidorf Eye Group at 818-883-0112 or through his Web site: **www.davidorf.com**.

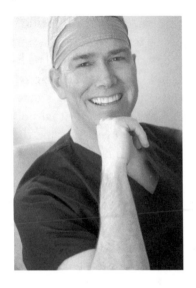

Robert K. Maloney, M.D., M.A. (Oxon), is a former Rhodes Scholar and Summa Cum Laude graduate of Harvard University. He completed his education at Oxford University and Johns Hopkins Hospital. Dr Maloney was the first surgeon in western North America to perform LASIK surgery as part of the original FDA clinical trials.

Dr. Maloney is perhaps best known as the exclusive LASIK surgeon on ABC's hit series *Extreme Makeover*. He has also been widely recognized by his peers, who voted him one of America's top 10 vision correction specialists in a nationwide survey conducted by *Ophthalmology Times*. He is the recipient of the prestigious 2001 Distinguished Lans Award, presented to one surgeon in the world by the International Society of Refractive Surgeons, for his innovative contributions to the field of vision correction surgery. The American Academy of Ophthalmology has awarded him the Senior Honor Award for contributions to the education of other eye surgeons and the Secretariat Award for distinguished contributions to the Academy.

Dr. Maloney is Clinical Professor of Ophthalmology at U.C.L.A and Director of the Maloney Vision Institute in West Los Angeles, California. He has trained more than 700 surgeons in the use of the excimer laser, and has personally performed more than 40,000 vision correction surgeries. He has published more than 100 articles, abstracts, and reports in professional journals and has delivered more than 200 invited lectures on five continents.

Dr. Maloney's research centers on developing new technologies for vision correction surgery, including the implantable contact lens and the light adjustable lens, and on complications of vision correction surgery. He has been a principal investigator for fourteen FDA clinical trials. He has a special clinic devoted to treating patients who have had problems with prior vision correction surgery.

He has been interviewed by The Discovery Channel, The Learning Channel, NBC's Extra, ABC's 20/20 and Prime Time Live, PBS's Life and Times, and CNN's The World Today. He has also been featured in numerous magazines and newspapers.

Dr. Maloney may be reached by calling the Maloney Vision Institute at 877-EYESIGHT or 310-208-3937, or he may be reached through his website: **www.maloneyvision.com**.